PHARMACOKINETICS AND ADVERSE EFFECTS OF DRUGS - MECHANISMS AND RISKS FACTORS

Edited by **Ntambwe Malangu**

Pharmacokinetics and Adverse Effects of Drugs - Mechanisms and Risks Factors

http://dx.doi.org/10.5772/intechopen.68518
Edited by Ntambwe Malangu

Contributors

Irmak Sayin Alan, Bahadir Alan, Maria Bogdan, Daniela Calina, Eliza Gofita, Adina Turcu-Stiolica, Anca Oana Docea, Adrian Camen, Gratiela Eliza Popa, Liliana Mititelu-Tartau, Gabriela Rusu, Ina Cristofor, Liliana Pavel, Tudor Adrian Balseanu, Yuki Murakami, Yukio Imamura, Pedro Amariles, Alejandra Cano-Paniagua, Calvin C.P. Pang, Kai On Chu, Katherine Dunnington, Nadia Cardillo Marricco, Christine Brandquist, Mike DiSpirito, Julie Grenier, Ntambwe Malangu

First published in London, United Kingdom, 2018 by IntechOpen
IntechOpen is the global imprint of INTECHOPEN LIMITED, registered in England and Wales, registration number: 11086078, The Shard, 25th floor, 32 London Bridge Street
London, SE19SG – United Kingdom
Printed in Croatia

British Library Cataloguing-in-Publication Data
A catalogue record for this book is available from the British Library

Additional hard copies can be obtained from orders@intechopen.com

Pharmacokinetics and Adverse Effects of Drugs - Mechanisms and Risks Factors, Edited by Ntambwe Malangu
p. cm.
Print ISBN 978-1-78923-138-0
Online ISBN 978-1-78923-139-7

For EU product safety concerns:
IN TECH d.o.o., Prolaz Marije Krucifikse Kozulić 3, 51000 Rijeka, Croatia,
info@intechopen.com or visit our website at intechopen.com.

Meet the editor

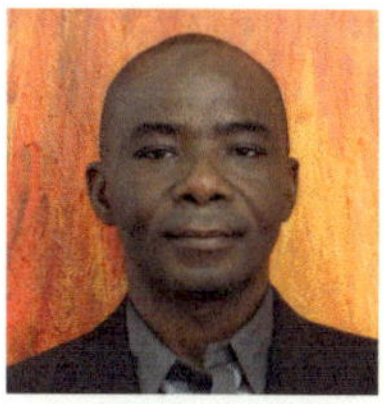

Prof. Ntambwe Malangu, born in Kabinda, Congo (DRC), is a pharmacoepidemiologist with public health expertise in drug safety issues. He is currently the Head of the Department of Epidemiology and Biostatistics at the School of Public Health at Sefako Makgatho Health Sciences University, Pretoria, South Africa; a Production Editor for *PULA: Botswana Journal for African Studies*; as well as a reviewer for a handful of international peer-reviewed journals. He has worked in both private and public sectors of the healthcare industry in several African countries. Since 2006, he has been working as an international health consultant and technical advisor with major development partners. In this capacity, he has contributed to several health system strengthening initiatives across the Anglophone, Lusophone, and Francophone African countries. He is a well-known trainer in supply chain management of health commodities and pharmaceuticals as well as in pharmacy and public health practice themes. Malangu holds a Bachelor's degree in Pharmacy from the University of Kinshasa (1991), a Master of Medical Science degree (Pharmacology and Toxicology) from the Medical University of Southern Africa (2003), a PhD degree (Pharmacoepidemiology and Pharmacovigilance) (2007), and a Doctor of Medical Sciences degree (Injury Epidemiology and Toxicovigilance) from the University of Limpopo (2012). Malangu has over 60 publications including scientific abstracts and letters, books, book chapters, and full papers.

Contents

Preface

Adverse effects as unwanted outcomes of drug effects occur generally when the upper threshold of therapeutic dosage range is reached. Several events and factors may lower this threshold or bring about the trespassing of the therapeutic level. The relevant events include what happens during the journey of the drug in the body, from its absorption from the site of administration, through its distribution and metabolism, to its elimination from the body. Every chapter in this book discusses and provides illustrations on the theme discussed based on authors' understanding and experience while summarizing existing knowledge. In doing so, each chapter provides a new insight that would benefit a novice as well as a seasoned reader in understanding the mechanisms and risk factors involved in the occurrence of adverse effects of drugs.

Chapter 1 explains the linkages between pharmacokinetic processes and the occurrence of adverse effects. It provides an overview on how through direct actions and interactions drugs produce changes in absorption, metabolism and transformation, distribution in organs, and elimination from the body. These changes as moderated by individual risk factors such as the genetic makeup, sociodemographic and health status, and lifestyle factors lead to the elicitation of adverse effects observed in clinical practice.

Chapter 2 dwells on the pharmacokinetics of one of the most common beverages worldwide, the green tea. This chapter elaborates on how food interactions affect the absorption of catechins and provides some practical illustrations that would help tea drinkers to maximize the benefits of this beverage. It further details how subsequent steps, namely, metabolism, distribution, and elimination, of the catechins take place in the mechanisms underlying these steps.

Chapter 3 illustrates the role of enzymatic transformations that result in the advent of depressive symptoms in patients suffering from chronic hepatitis C treated with interferon alpha (IFN-α). In this chapter, the findings presented demonstrate how upward changes in concentration in plasma and in other compartments such as in cerebrospinal fluid of tryptophan (TRP)-kynurenine (KYN) and its active metabolites [3-hydroxykynurenine (3-HK), kynurenic acid (KA), and quinolinic acid (QUIN)] are associated with the severity of depressive symptoms clinically seen as adverse effects of IFN-α. This chapter links up to the first chapter in making an exposé of one of the mechanisms by which pharmacokinetic processes lead to the advent of adverse effects.

Chapter 4 shows the major roles of pharmacokinetics in drug development, particularly how pharmacokinetic data are useful in ascertaining the safety profile of drugs under development. It provides technical details of relevant steps and endpoints for each phase of a drug development; in doing so, the chapter demonstrates how pharmacokinetic studies are an important tool used to link exposure to efficacy and safety and how they assist in determining the dosages of marketed drugs.

Chapter 5 provides an overview on hepatotoxicity of drugs: how several drugs affect the organ that is responsible for most of the metabolism in the body, the liver. It is noted that metabolism is a key step that achieves two major objectives: firstly, in transforming a non-active substance or prodrug into active metabolites, it helps in the elicitation of the pharmacodynamic action of the drug, and, secondly, in transforming an active drug into inactive hydrosoluble metabolites, it helps in facilitating the elimination of the drug from the body, thereby preventing accumulation that may result in unwanted or adverse effects. This chapter proposes an approach and a scale that could be used for identifying liver toxicity.

Chapter 6 describes the side effects of glucocorticoids; this chapter illustrates how some drugs produce several adverse effects that affect several organs and systems in the body. Glucocorticoids are a classic example of how the usefulness of certain drugs is counterbalanced by high risks associated with their use. The sheer extent of the range of side and adverse effects from glucocorticoids is a reminder on how narrow the therapeutic window is and why clinicians and patients should be vigilant in monitoring untoward effects of drugs.

Chapter 7 provides an update on the side effects of new antidepressants. Having been hailed as better than the old antidepressants, this review on new antidepressants demonstrates how pharmacokinetic parameters played an important role in the discovery of some of these new antidepressants and also how they affect the spread of adverse effects.

As a whole, this book, as a fruit from the collaborative work from several international scientists, will be a useful resource for researchers, students, and clinicians. Each individual chapter could serve as a prescribed reading for postgraduate students and clinicians specializing in and practicing clinical pharmacology and toxicology, pharmacotherapy and pharmacotherapeutics, pharmacovigilance, and toxicovigilance, as well as those involved in clinical research, drug discovery, and development.

It is with a heart full of gratitude that I present to you the team of international scientists who contributed to this volume: Drs. Katherine Dunnington, Natacha Benrimoh, Christine Brandquist, Nadia Cardillo-Marricco, Mike Di Spirito, and Julie Grenier from Celerion, a premier Clinical Research Organization, Nebraska, USA; Dr. Kai On Chu and Prof. Calvin Pang from the Chinese University of Hong Kong; Dr. Yuki Murakami from Doshisha University, Kyoto, Japan, and Dr. Yukio Imamura from Osaka University Graduate School of Medicine, Japan; Irmak Sayın Alan and Bahadır Alan from the Medical Faculty of Okan University, Istanbul, Turkey; Alejandra Cano Paniagua and Pedro Amariles from the Research Group on Pharmaceutical Prevention and Promotion, University of Antioquia, Colombia; and Drs. Maria Bogdan, Eliza Gofita, Daniela Cornelia Calina, Adina Turcu-Stiolica, Anca Oana Docea, Tudor Adrian Balseanu, Adrian Camen, Gratiela Eliza Popa, Gabriela Rusu, Ina Cristofor, Liliana Pavel, and Liliana Mititelu-Tartau from the University of Medicine and Pharmacy (Craiova, Galati, and Iasi) in Romania.

Finally, I thank and pass the baton to my three sons, David, Daniel, and Miraciel, whose quality time was diverted to edit this book. Furthermore, I salute and acknowledge the major role played by Marina Dusevic as well as the publishing, production, and editorial teams from IntechOpen®.

Professor Ntambwe Malangu
Sefako Makgatho Health Sciences University
Pretoria, South Africa

Chapter 1

Introductory Chapter: Linkages between Pharmacokinetics and Adverse Effects of Drugs

Ntambwe Malangu

Additional information is available at the end of the chapter

http://dx.doi.org/10.5772/intechopen.76511

1. Introduction

This chapter aims to elaborate on the linkages between pharmacokinetics and the advent of adverse effects of drugs. It is well known that pharmacokinetics is about the journey of the drug in the body, from its absorption, through its distribution and metabolism, to its elimination from the body. During this journey, after its absorption and distribution, the drug reaches its specific sites where it interacts with its receptors, usually proteins and enzymes, and produces its biological effects; this is known as "pharmacodynamics." The biological effects lead to clinical effects that are observed in patients; this is known as "therapeutics or pharmacotherapeutics." In the following sections, the actions of the body on a drug and the actions of the drug on the body are reviewed in each stage to explain how adverse effects occur. In doing so, the mechanisms and risk factors of adverse effects will be addressed. The next section deals with the absorption, followed by the distribution and excretion of drugs as they relate to the occurrence of adverse effects. A final section will deal with risk factors before some concluding remarks are presented.

2. Rates of absorption influence on the occurrence of adverse effects

For the majority of drugs that are administered by other routes than intravenous injection, they need to overcome several hurdles before they reach the systemic circulation. These include the layers of the outer skin of the body or veins in case of subcutaneous and intramuscular routes or the walls of the digestive system. For drugs administered orally, the active substances must first be released from the dosage from, namely tablets, capsules, and other forms. There will be a reduction of therapeutic effects if there is little absorption, or destruction of the drug by digestive system enzymes, or if the active substance was not released from its dosage form [1, 2]. Sometimes the absorption may be impaired by the presence of foods or other drugs or substances that react with the active substance and make it not absorbable. On the contrary, the presence of physical lesions in the digestive tract, or substances that increases the liposolubility of the active substance may actually increase its absorption [3].

Several factors affect the journey of the drug that result in increased or decreased absorption or volume of distribution as well as the metabolism thereof. The physicochemical characteristics of the drug itself, the pharmaceutical dosage form it is in and its intrinsic quality, the state of the first layers of skin or membranes through which the drug is to be absorbed through, the composition of the environment such as the presence or absence of foods or other chemicals in the digestive system as well as the type of foods or the other chemicals, the type and number of carriers subunits of enzymes or proteins complex available at the site of absorption, all influence the absorption rates [4].

For medicines administered orally, whether tablets, capsules, solution, suspension, syrup, or elixir, it should be noted that the gastrointestinal tract is a harsh environment. With its low pH, acid-labile drugs such as benzylpenicillin (penicillin G) and methicillin, they become inactivated as a result of the catalysis that takes place due to beta-lactamase enzymes [4–6]. Similarly, the presence of proteases makes the oral route unsuitable for many proteins and peptides such as insulin and oxytocin [1–3]. When taken orally, the absorption of drugs occurs chiefly by passive diffusion of lipophilic molecules and by carrier-mediated transport for drugs that are structurally similar to endogenous compounds such as levodopa and 5-fluorouracil. With passive diffusion, the rate of absorption is proportional to the concentration or the amount of drug to be absorbed and the fraction or percentage absorbed in a given interval remains constant.

With carrier-mediated mechanisms, be it active transport or facilitated diffusion, there is a limited capacity and the transporter can be saturated, hence limiting the amount of drug reaching the systemic circulation. In this instance, increasing the dose will result in local adverse effects [6]. Clinicians ought to understand the particularity of a particular drug before deciding to indiscriminately increase the dose when a subtherapeutic effect is observed. Indeed, this remark is true even for drugs absorbed by passive diffusion like aspirin (salicylic acid) as the percentage absorbed is independent of the continuous concentration but proportional to the initial drug concentration.

Nowadays, the proliferation of substandard and falsified drugs particularly in Africa makes it difficult to predict the beneficial effects of these drugs [7]. This is because the intrinsic pharmaceutical quality of these drugs is not optimal leading to several consequences with regard to the absorption and elicited effects of these drugs. Several examples have been encountered in clinical practice; for instance, cotrimoxazole tablets badly compressed have been taken by patients just to be excreted intact in their feces! This example means that no dissolution took place, so little or nothing of the drug was absorbed, consequently, the therapeutic effects expected from the drug could not be elicited rather than the placebo effect.

As depicted in **Figure 1**, largely unionized substances such as, aspirin when in acidic environment, it is absorbed from the stomach but most of the absorption occurs in the small intestine where the large surface area compensates for the less favorable degree of ionization. On the contrary, weak bases, which are highly ionized in gastric acid, cannot be absorbed until they have left the stomach, so delayed gastric emptying (when foods is in the stomach) can delay the effect of such drugs [6, 8].

On the other hand, it is often recommended that drugs should be taken at meal times. This is to aid adherence to treatment and in some circumstances, to reduce gastric irritation (a local adverse effect), as, for example, with aspirin, which may cause gastric bleeding. It is noted here that the effect of food is not always predictable, although, generally, food delays gastric emptying and increases the secretion of gastric acid while reducing the overall gastric pH. Hence, the presence of foods may reduce the absorption of drugs such as ketoconazole that are more soluble in acid; yet on the contrary, the absorption of griseofulvin, an antifungal drug, as well as that of saquinavir, an antiretroviral drug, is increased when taken with a "fatty" meal [6, 9, 10].

As depicted in **Figure 2**, several transportation mechanisms have been envisaged from the site of absorption. It should be noted that the preponderance of each transport mechanism is different for each individual patient due to their genetic and constitutional makeup.

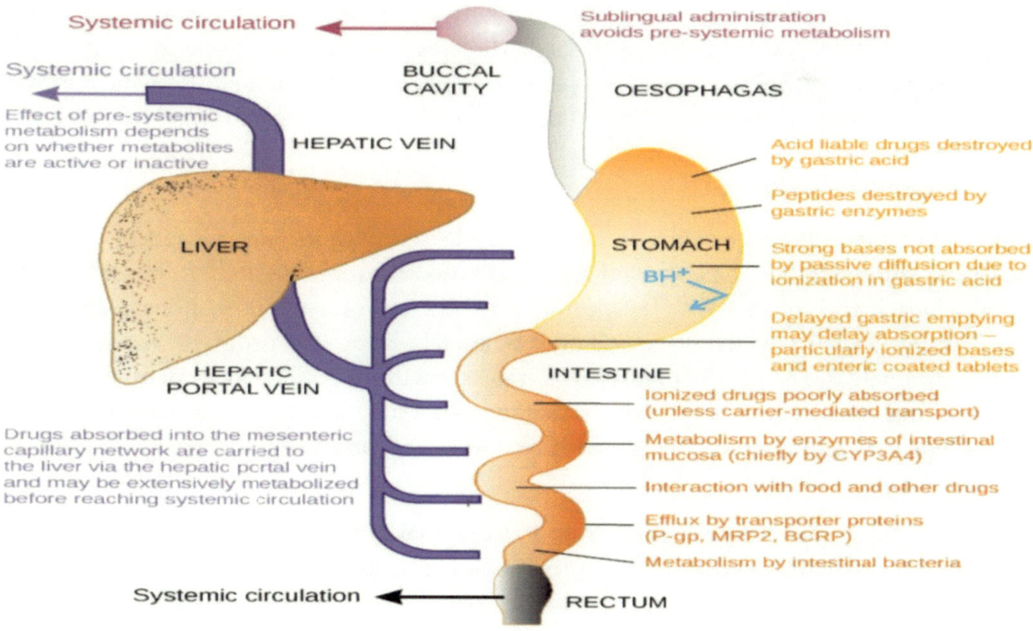

Figure 1. Absorption throughout the gastrointestinal tract. Source: [6].

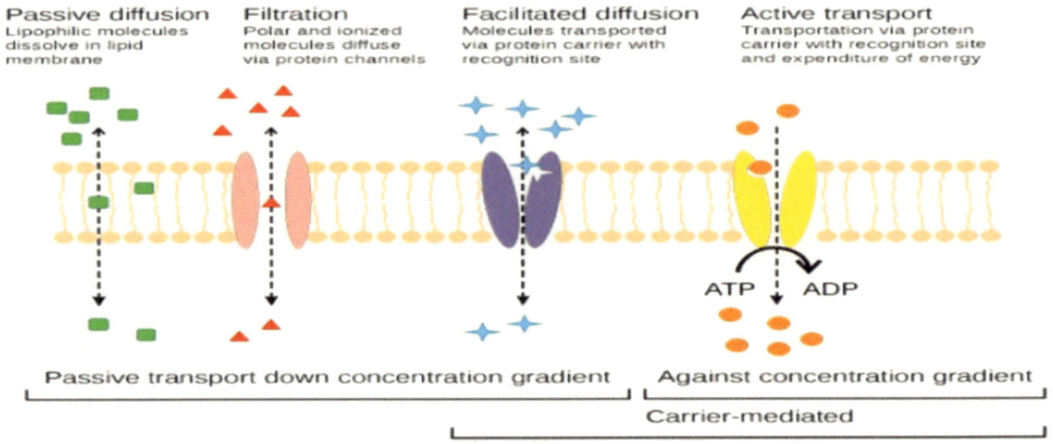

Figure 2. Transport mechanisms of drugs. Source: [6].

3. Systemic concentration and occurrence of adverse effects

The key concept in explaining the effects of drugs is "plasma concentration" or the amount of drug that reaches the systematic circulation; it reflects the amount of drug that will be available to act and produce effects at the site of action. Classically, it is has been established that what is known as the effect of a drug is actually a combination of the action of a drug or drug action; its effect or drug effect and the body's response or drug response. This may be illustrated as follows: For example, for a penicillin antibiotic, the "action" consists of inhibiting bacterial protein synthesis, the "effect" corresponds to the killing rate or growth inhibition rate of bacteria, and the clinical "response" would be the cure of the body from the infection and its manifestations [6, 11, 12].

In order to achieve its effect, a drug must first be released from its pharmaceutical form from the site of administration; be absorbed and distributed through the body to reach its site of action where it will interact with its specific receptors and/or some other nonspecific receptors. Through its journey, the body acts on it by metabolizing it in order, primarily, to wear off and eliminate it. The result of metabolism may sometimes achieve the goal of inactivating or destroying the structure of the drug; or sometimes it may lead to the production of active metabolites that actually will interact with receptors and produce the expected therapeutic effects of the particular drug [11, 13, 14].

For drugs subject the first-pass effect that is drugs that are metabolized before they reach the systemic circulation; generally, this pre-systemic metabolism reduces their bioavailability except when and if the resulting metabolites are pharmacologically active. In the case of nitroglycerin, which is almost totally first metabolized, its di- and mononitrate metabolites produced have very much reduced activity, and hence this drug is considered to be inactive when taken orally [15].

When a drug successfully crosses the physical and biochemical barriers described above, it will reach the systemic circulation and its plasma concentration will continue to rise as for as it will be absorbed. If, the increase is beyond a certain threshold, toxic effects or adverse effects will be clinically observed. This is well established now that there is an optimum range of concentrations over which a drug has beneficial or expected useful effects, with no clinical toxicity, this is known as the "therapeutic range," sometimes referred to as the "therapeutic window" [6]. Moreover, it has been established also that there is a threshold concentration below which the drug is deemed ineffective, or not producing expected therapeutics effects, and a higher threshold above which adverse or unwanted toxic effects become apparent as shown in **Figure 3**.

The plasma concentration fluctuates based on the rates of absorption, the influence of the first-pass effect, and based on whether the drug is following a one compartment model of distribution or a multiple compartment model. For drugs using the multiple compartment model, which are drugs that accumulate in other compartments other than the systemic circulation, namely the liver, skeletal muscles, bones, adipose tissues; their absorption, distribution, and metabolism may be complex. For instance, thiopental, once absorbed, its liver concentrations rapidly equilibrate with those in plasma while the concentrations in skeletal muscle rise initially and then equilibrate later and their concentrations in adipose tissue will rise for at least the first 3.5 h following the bolus injection of thiopental; its duration of action will be short due to uptake of the drug into skeletal muscle and fat [16–18].

In order to understand the influence of multiple compartments, it is important to remember that typically the body is made of 11 chemical elements, namely carbon, calcium, chlorine, hydrogen, nitrogen, magnesium, oxygen, phosphorus, potassium, sodium, and sulfur; and 5 molecules such as water which comprises 60–62%; proteins 16–18%; fat 10–15%; minerals 6–7%; up to 1% of carbohydrates [19, 20] (**Figure 4**).

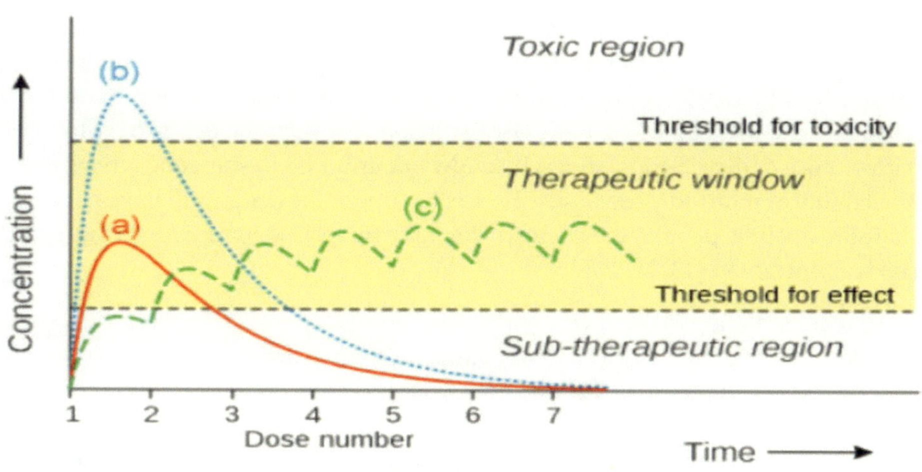

Figure 3. Drug levels in relation to elicited effects. Source: [6].

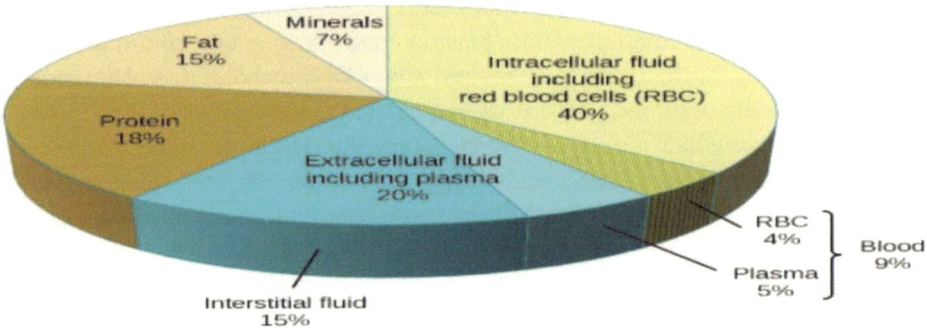

Figure 4. Body composition. Source: Fomon et al. [19]; Chumlea et al. [20].

It should be noted that there are variations in the concentration of the elements and molecules making up the body. These variations are rhythmic, cyclic, and dependent on the age, sex, and health status of the individuals. It is known that, in each disease state, and in case of multi-morbidity, the composition of these elements and molecules vary in relation to the lifestyle of an individual, namely his/her water and food intake, smoking and alcohol consumption, exercise and sleeping patterns in terms of quantity, quality, and variety or diversity [21–24]. This situation largely explains why a same dose of a drug may not always produce similar effects (beneficial or adverse) on a group of individuals even if they have same bodyweights, are of same ethnicity or sex. This observation explains why standard doses cannot be prescribed indiscriminately to each individual patient; hence the new concept of individualized treatment regimen.

The need for individualized regimen can be more understood when one considers the "half-life" concept. Half-life is a very useful parameter in pharmacokinetics; it is defined as the time it takes for the concentration of a drug to halve from its initial peak concentration in plasma or urine. It is important to note that even drugs from the same class have different half-lives because they have different volumes of distribution and/or systemic clearance. This is so because the apparent volume of distribution depends, as said earlier, upon the nature of the drug and the makeup of individuals. For instance, lipophilic drugs tend to have large apparent volumes of distribution and to be widely distributed in someone who is obese, due to the availability of more adipose tissue. Hence, the lipophilic drugs will have a longer elimination half-life in obese people; their longer stay may mean also longer lingering affects both beneficial and unwanted [23, 25, 26].

When drugs accumulating in other compartments continue to be taken, there will be a saturation of the receptors or even storage spaces in these compartments, resulting in much more concentrations in the interstitial liquids, and overwhelming of related receptors, thus the advent of adverse and side effects not typical of drug class. Such side effects may and should become a subject of pharmacovigilance investigation. It should be said here that atypical or new side effects may occur even with normal doses in certain individuals because of their uniqueness with regard to the receptors, enzymes, or proteins, they may have in abundance or absence thereof as a matter of their genetic makeup or as a result of a subclinical or clinical disease state as well as their lifestyle as already explained. In case of overdose, drug metabolism is altered because enzymes responsible for metabolism become saturated; this leaves the excess drug free to force its way to nonspecific receptors by overcoming both inhibition or competition; consequently, it produces nontypical adverse effects while its clearance is decreased and its half-life is prolonged [27–30].

4. Elimination or excretion of drugs and adverse effects

Once a drug is metabolized and reduced to hydrosoluble entities, it is ready to be excreted through the kidneys and eliminated in the urine. However, some changes may impact negatively to this process. An important pharmacokinetic change in the elderly, for instance, is the decrease in renal drug elimination due to the fact that as someone ages, his/her renal mass as well as glomerular filtration and tubular secretion capacities decrease. It should be noted that after age 40, there is a decrease in the number of functional glomeruli, and the renal blood flow is estimated to decline by approximately 1% yearly. The clinical effect of decreased renal clearance includes prolonged drug half-life, increased serum drug level to toxic level which obviously leads to increased potential for adverse drug reactions [6, 31].

5. Pharmacokinetics related risk factors of adverse effects

At the core, genetic factors play a major role because of the genetic polymorphism or difference in drug responses between individuals. The drug response is genetically determined by the type, quality, and quantity of genes, proteins, enzymes that one has. A well-known example suffices here, the case of the enzyme, N-acetyltransferase which differs between individuals such that the population may be divided into slow and fast acetylators. People who are slow acetylators may experience more adverse effects unless doses of drugs requiring acetylation for metabolism are reduced. Other inherited variations in pharmacokinetics include deficiency of one or more hepatic cytochrome-P450 isozymes or plasma cholinesterase enzymes. The metabolic conversion of drugs into metabolites is established as a source of several idiosyncratic drug reactions [32–38].

As stated above, lifestyle factors such as diet and exercise affect bodyweight which is used as the basis for determining the dose administered. In case of chronic diseases, an increase or a drop of 10–20% in bodyweight should normally be noted and followed by a dose adjustment. Tuberculosis treatment is an example whereby patients normally increase their bodyweights sometimes up to 30% of their initial weights within 2–4 months. Clearly based on the treatment algorithms as defined by WHO, the doses or number of tablets for these patients should increase following the increase in their bodyweights; however, often this is not usually done [39, 40]. Moreover, diet, smoking, and alcohol may affect enzyme activity and lead to unexpected drug interactions. Cigarette smoking affects drug therapy by pharmacokinetic. The polycyclic aromatic hydrocarbons in tobacco smoke are believed to be responsible for the induction of cytochrome P450 (CYP) 1A1 and CYP1A2 which are responsible for the metabolism of a number of drugs. Drugs for which induced metabolism because of cigarette smoking may have clinical consequence include theophylline, caffeine, tacrine, imipramine, haloperidol, pentazocine, propranolol, flecainide, and estradiol. Cigarette smoking results in faster clearance of heparin, possibly related to smoking-related activation of thrombosis that results in enhanced heparin binding to antithrombin factor III [41, 42]. Moreover, cutaneous vasoconstriction by nicotine may slow the rate of insulin absorption after subcutaneous administration. Hence, the impact of cigarette smoking needs to be considered in planning and assessing responses to drug therapy; this why clinicians should regularly enquire of smoking and drinking habits of their patients [43, 44].

With regard to sex, differences between male and female will include differences in weight and weight distribution as well as hormonal differences particularly in relation to the menstrual cycle and its absence in prepubescent girls and postmenopausal women [45]. Moreover, physiological differences relating to body composition, gastric motility, liver metabolism, renal function, and glomerular filtration rates all affect differently the disposition of drugs with regard to gender. Simply put, drug absorption, distribution, metabolism, and elimination are not actually similar in men and women. Drug absorption in the lung may differ according to gender [46]. It has been demonstrated that there is a significant less deposition of an aerosolized drug in women than men which has been ascribed to differences in breathing patterns. Gastrointestinal transit time is longer in women (mean 91.7 h) than in men (44.8 h), as is gastric emptying time. This situation causes delays in the absorption of certain drugs. It has been shown for instance that following oral doses of levofloxacin and losartan, the areas under the curve (AUC) of these drugs were significantly greater in females than males. Moreover, relatively fast absorption of oral salicylates and that of ferrous sulfate has been shown in females and prepubertal girls than in boys. After intravenous infusion, the systemic clearance of verapamil was shown to be greater in women than in men. In case of propofol, women are said to be less sensitive to the effects of propofol and recover from anesthesia more quickly than men. This observation was demonstrated in a study that showed that the AUC values for the metabolites, 4-hydroxypropofol and propofol glucuronide, were significantly higher in women than in men and that this effect was 3.6 times higher in Hispanic females than in Caucasian females. On the contrary, protein binding is reportedly higher in males than females, for chlordiazepoxide and warfarin. Hepatic enzyme CYP3A4 is more active in females than males; drugs metabolized by this enzyme are thus affected more efficiently in females than males [47–50].

With regard to age, in children, their low gastric acid secretion can result in increased serum concentrations of weak bases and acid-labile medications, such as penicillin, and decreased serum concentrations of weak acid medications, such as phenobarbital, due to increased ionization. Additionally, gastric emptying time and intestinal transit time are delayed in premature infants; this increases drug contact time with the GI mucosa, hereby increasing drug absorption. In neonates, infants, and young children, there is increased risk of ADRs because of their incapacity to metabolize most drugs due to lack of appropriate enzymes and related functions. For instance, in neonates of less than 2 months old, because of their immature renal tubular function, it is recommended to avoid digoxin, aminoglycosides, ACE inhibitors, and NSAIDs [11, 51–53].

In the elderly, it is well known that the incidence of diseases increases with aging. A major consideration is the presence of comorbid conditions present in aging people that affect plasma concentrations of drugs through changes in the extent of absorption, in the rates of metabolism and/or excretion, and changes in tissue localization, for example, increased tissue binding leading to reduced plasma concentrations. In case of warfarin, age was found to have a significant effect on dosing; older patients require much lower doses than the young adults. Furthermore, it is well established that higher gastric pH, delayed gastric emptying, and decreased intestinal motility and blood flow are observed in elderly individuals. Consequently, even normal doses for health adults may become overdosage in the elderly patients who may experience more and severe adverse effects. Other factors that affect distribution of drugs in the body are changes in body fat and water and changes in protein binding. In the elderly, lean body mass can decrease by as much as 12–19% through the loss of skeletal muscle. Thus, blood levels of drugs primarily distributed in muscle such as digoxin will increase and become a risk for overdose when normal or standard dose are used. Moreover, due to a decrease in water concentration in older people, hydrosoluble drugs would reach higher concentrations because there is less water to dilute them while liposoluble drugs would accumulate more because there is relatively more fat tissue to store them. Furthermore, the kidney and liver functions perform less optimally; hence drugs are not readily metabolized and excreted into the urine to be eliminated. This leads to many drugs staying much longer than they do in a younger person's body, the net result would be the prolongation of pharmacodynamic effects and occurrence of side effects [2, 54–63].

With regard to disease states, there are pharmacodynamic differences in patients with liver disease. Effects have been observed with β-blockers and drugs that depress the CNS. In case of β-blockers, it is documented that there is a reduction in β-adrenoceptor density in mononuclear cells which results in a decrease in effect; this has been observed with propranolol. Similarly, patients with liver cirrhosis had been found to be particularly sensitive to opioids and anxiolytics. In case of kidney disease, a drug that is 100% metabolized may also be affected to some extent particularly its excretion if its metabolites accumulate in plasma, leading to an exaggerated response if the metabolites contribute to the pharmacological effect; or, atypical toxicity that is not seen when the metabolites are excreted normally. Additionally, renal impairment is likely to lead to varying degrees of water loading and this may lead to the changes in the concentrations of the drug in the fluid compartments of the body, including plasma. Children with cystic fibrosis present with greater renal clearance of drugs such as aminoglycosides when compared with children without the disease; this observation suggests that higher doses by weight and more frequent dosing intervals are required in these children [64–72].

With regard to drug-drug interactions, it should be said that patients commonly use two or more drugs concurrently; some prescribed by their health care providers, others bought by themselves or received from family and friends. Because patients are often unaware of the multiple drug interactions, they suffer from adverse drug reactions resulting from alterations of the pharmacokinetics parameters due to interacting substances; often with the end result being a decreased therapeutic efficacy, or an increased toxicity or occurrence of adverse effects. The binding of drugs to macromolecules such as receptors on plasma proteins is governed by the law of mass action which states that "the rate at which a chemical reaction proceeds is proportional to the active masses (usually molar concentrations) of the reacting substances." Taken from chemistry point of view, this concept means that for the reaction to occur, collision between the reacting molecules must take place. It follows that the rate of reaction will be proportional to the number of collisions; while the number of collisions will be proportional to the molar concentrations of the reacting molecules. Hence, drugs-foods and drugs-drugs interactions will affect the rates of a drug disposition based on the quantities available of the doses taken and the synchronicity which implies the presence of both substances at the same time for them to interact directly or indirectly through competition or inhibition of relevant receptors. The above observations imply that the degree of drug interaction depends on the relative concentrations of each drug; hence, the dose and the time of administration are critical elements in the onset of adverse effects resulting from drug-drug interactions. These interactions may produce changes in absorption rate, competition for binding sites on plasma proteins, oral bioavailability, extent and volume of distribution in organs and tissues, and hepatic and renal clearance as well as the extent of elimination from the body. Indeed besides other medicines, drugs of abuse, herbal medicines, and foodstuffs have been reported to affect the pharmacokinetics of specific drugs [73–78].

The above observations suggest the need for caution when prescribing more than one drug as well as the need to counsel patients about the dangers of taking nonprescribed drugs, drugs for entertainment including alcoholic drinks without seeking proper advice from health care professionals [79–84].

6. Concluding remarks

Adverse effects as unwanted outcomes of drugs effects occur generally when the upper threshold of therapeutic dosage range is reached. However, several factors may lower this threshold or bring about the trespassing of the therapeutic level. Risks factors include intrinsic properties of the drugs and the pharmaceutical dosage forms issues and interactions that affect their pharmacokinetics as well as the sociodemographic, health status, and lifestyle factors superimposed on the genetic makeup of a person. Clinicians ought to understand the pharmacokinetics of a drug before deciding to adjust dosages particularly upwardly as a precautionary measure to preempt dose-related adverse effects. Equally, they should not refrain from doing so when the situation warrants it; such as when the bodyweights of patients have significantly increased or when pharmacokinetic changes dictate so.

Author details

Ntambwe Malangu

Address all correspondence to: gustavmalangu@gmail.com

School of Public Health, Sefako Makgatho Health Sciences University, South Africa

References

[1] Alomar MJ. Factors affecting the development of adverse drug reactions. SaudI Pharmaceutical Journal. 2014;**22**(2):83-94

[2] Anderson BJ, Holford NH. Mechanism-based concepts of size and maturity in pharmacokinetics. Annual Review of Pharmacology and Toxicology. 2008;**48**:303-332

[3] Yang Z. The roles of membrane transporters on the oral drug absorption. Journal of Molecular Pharmaceutics and Organic Process Research. 2013;**1**:e102

[4] Shugarts S, Benet LZ. The role of transporters in the pharmacokinetics of orally administered drugs. Pharmaceutical Research. 2009;**26**:2039-2054

[5] Derendorf H, Hochhaus G, editors. Handbook of Pharmacokinetic/Pharmacodynamic Correlation. Boca Raton, FL: CRC Press; 1995

[6] Curry SH, Whelpton R. Introduction to Drug Disposition and Pharmacokinetics. 1st ed. UK: John Wiley & Sons, Ltd; 2017

[7] Malangu N. Risks associated with international trading of medicines by non-licensed entities and non-professionals. In: Macek A, editor. International Trade-on the Brink of Change. InTech; 2017. ISBN-978-953-51-2912-7

[8] Wasan KM, Brocks DR, Lee SD, Sachs-Barrable K, Thronton SJ. Impact of lipoproteins on the biological activity and disposition of hydrophobic drugs: Implications for drug discovery. Nature Reviews. Drug Discovery. 2008;**7**:84-99

[9] Müller F, Fromm MF. Transporter-mediated drug-drug interactions. Pharmacogenomics. 2011;**12**:1017-1037

[10] Johnson TN, Thomson M. Intestinal metabolism and transport of drugs in children: The effects of age and disease. Journal of Pediatric Gastroenterology and Nutrition. 2008;**47**:3-10

[11] De-gregori S, Ranzani GN, Borghesi A, Regazzi M, Stronati M. Drug transporters and renal drug disposition in the newborn. The Journal of Maternal-Fetal & Neonatal Medicine. 2009;**22**:31-37

[12] Beer J, Wagner CC, Zeitlinger M. Protein binding of antimicrobials: Methods for quantification and for investigation of its impact on bacterial killing. The AAPS Journal. 2009;**11**(1):1

[13] Amdur MO, Doull J, Klaassen CD, editors. Casarett and Doull's Toxicology: The Basic Science of Poisons. Elmsford, NY: Pergamon Press; 1991

[14] Starner CI, Gray SL, Guay DR, et al. Geriatrics. In: DiPiro JT, Talbert RL, Yee GC, et al., editors. Pharmacotherapy: A Pathophysiologic Approach. 7th ed. New York, NY: McGraw-Hill; 2008. pp. 57-66

[15] Kitteringham NR, Park BK, Pirmohamed M. The role of active metabolites in drug toxicity. Drug Safety. 1994;**11**:114-144

[16] Barre J, Houin G, Rosenbaum J, Zini R, Dhumeaux D, Tillement JP. Decreased alpha 1-acid glycoprotein in liver cirrhosis: Consequences for drug protein binding. British Journal of Clinical Pharmacology. 1984;**18**:652-653

[17] Anderson SG, Livingston M, Couchman L, Smith DJ, Connolly M, Miller J, et al. Sex differences in plasma clozapine and norclozapine concentrations in clinical practice and in relation to body mass index and plasma glucose concentrations: A retrospective survey. Annals of General Psychiatry. 2015;**14**(1):39

[18] Routledge PA, Stargel WW, Kitchell BB. Sex-related differences in the plasma protein binding of lignocaine and diazepam. British Journal of Clinical Pharmacology. 1991;**11**:245-250

[19] Fomon SJ, Haschke F, Ziegler EE, Nelson SE. Body composition of reference children from birth to age 10 years. The American Journal of Clinical Nutrition. 1982;**35**:1169-1175

[20] Chumlea WC, Guo SS, Zeller CM, Reo NV, Siervogel RM. Total body water data for white adults 18 to 64 years of age: The Fels longitudinal study. Kidney International. 1999;**56**:244-252

[21] Aguilar-Roblero R. Chronostasis: The timing of physiological systems. In: Mechanisms of Circadian Systems in Animals and Their Clinical Relevance. Springer International Publishing; 2015. pp. 221-236

[22] Backman JT, Filppula AM, Niemi M, Neuvonen PJ. Role of cytochrome P450 2C8 in drug metabolism and interactions. Pharmacological Reviews. 2016;**68**(1):168-241

[23] Bern M, Sand KMK, Nilsen J, Sandlie I, Andersen JT. The role of albumin receptors in regulation of albumin homeostasis: Implications for drug delivery. Journal of Controlled Release. 2015;**211**:144-162

[24] Kuebler WM. Tides of blood: Cyclic changes in lung blood volume during a single breath. American Journal of Respiratory Cell and Molecular Biology. 2017;**57**(4):386-387

[25] Jahn A, Bodreau C, Farthing K, Elbarbry F. Assessing Propylene Glycol Toxicity in Alcohol Withdrawal Patients Receiving Intravenous Benzodiazepines: A One-Compartment Pharmacokinetic Model. European Journal of Drug Metabolism and Pharmacokinetics 2018:1-8

[26] Shao J, Kraft JC, Li B, Yu J, Freeling J, Koehn J, Ho RJ. Nanodrug formulations to enhance HIV drug exposure in lymphoid tissues and cells: Clinical significance and potential impact on treatment and eradication of HIV/AIDS. Nanomedicine. 2016;**11**(5):545-564

[27] Dartois V. The path of anti-tuberculosis drugs: From blood to lesions to mycobacterial cells. Nature Reviews Microbiology. 2014;**12**(3):159-167

[28] Zhitomirsky B, Assaraf YG. Lysosomal accumulation of anticancer drugs triggers lysosomal exocytosis. Oncotarget. 2017;**8**(28):45117-45132

[29] Srinivas N, Maffuid K, Kashuba AD. Clinical pharmacokinetics and pharmacodynamics of drugs in the central nervous system. Clinical Pharmacokinetics. 2018:1-16

[30] Jusko WJ. Clarification of contraceptive drug pharmacokinetics in obesity. Contraception. 2017;**95**(1):10-16

[31] Ritter J, Lionel L, Timothy M, Albert F. A Textbook of Clinical Pharmacology and Therapeutics. CRC Press; 2008

[32] Daly AK. Using genome-wide association studies to identify genes important in serious adverse drug reactions. Annual Review of Pharmacology and Toxicology. 2012;**52**:21-35

[33] Pirmohamed M, Park BK. Genetic susceptibility to adverse drug reactions. Trends in Pharmacological Sciences. 2001;**22**(6):298-305

[34] Falzon D, Holger JS, Elizabeth H, Licé GA, Christian L, Ernesto J, Karin W. World Health Organization treatment guidelines for drug-resistant tuberculosis, 2016 update. European Respiratory Journal. 2017;**49**(3):1602308

[35] U.S. Department of Health and Human Services. Health Consequences of Smoking: A Report of the Surgeon General [Internet]. Atlanta, GA: U.S.: Department of Health and Human Services, Centers for Disease Control and Prevention, National Center for Chronic Disease Prevention and Health Promotion, Office on Smoking and Health; 2004 [cited 2011 Oct 20]. Available from: http://www.surgeongeneral.gov/library/Smokingconsequences/

[36] van Hassselt JC, Iyengar R. Systems pharmacology-based identification of pharmacogenomic determinants of adverse drug reactions using human iPSC-derived cell lines. Current Opinion in Systems Biology. 2017;**4**:9-15

[37] Chung WH, Chang WC, Lee YS, Wu YY, Yang CH, Ho HC, et al. Genetic variants associated with phenytoin-related severe cutaneous adverse reactions. JAMA. 2014;**312**(5):525-534

[38] Crews KR, Gaedigk A, Dunnenberger HM, Leeder JS, Klein TE, Caudle KE, et al. Clinical Pharmacogenetics implementation consortium guidelines for cytochrome P450 2D6 genotype and codeine therapy: 2014 update. Clinical Pharmacology & Therapeutics. 2014;**95**(4):376-382

[39] World Health Organization. WHO Treatment Guidelines for Drug-Resistant Tuberculosis 2016 Update. World Health Organization; 2016

[40] Zumla A, Chakaya J, Centis R, D'Ambrosio L, Mwaba P, Bates M, et al. Tuberculosis treatment and management—An update on treatment regimens, trials, new drugs, and adjunct therapies. The Lancet Respiratory Medicine. 2015;**3**(3):220-234

[41] Verbeeck RK, Günther G, Kibuule D, Hunter C, Rennie TW. Optimizing treatment outcome of first-line anti-tuberculosis drugs: The role of therapeutic drug monitoring. European Journal of Clinical Pharmacology. 2016;**72**(8):905-916

[42] S Z, Benowitz NL. Drug interactions with tobacco smoking-An update. Clinical Pharmacokinetics. 1999;**36**(6):425-438

[43] Himmelmann A, Jendle J, Mellen A. The impact of smoking on inhaled insulin. Diabetes Care. 2003;**26**:677-682

[44] Taghavi T, Helen GS, Benowitz NL, Tyndale RF. Effect of UGT2B10, UGT2B17, FMO3, and OCT2 genetic variation on nicotine and cotinine pharmacokinetics and smoking in African Americans. Pharmacogenetics and Genomics. 2017;**27**(4):143-154

[45] Mitchell SC, Smith RL, Waring RH. The menstrual cycle and drug metabolism. Current Drug Metabolism. 2009;**10**(5):499-507

[46] Ofotokun I, Pomeroy C. Sex differences in adverse reactions to antiretroviral drugs. Topics in HIV Medicine. 2003;**11**(2):55-59

[47] Ensom M. Gender-based differences and menstrual cycle-related changes in specific diseases: Implications for pharmacotherapy. Pharmacotherapy. 2000;**20**(5):523-539

[48] Rodenburg EM, Stricker BH, Visser LE. Sex differences in cardiovascular drug-induced adverse reactions causing hospital admissions. British Journal of Clinical Pharmacology. 2012;**74**(6):1045-1052

[49] El-Eraky H, Thomas SHL. Effects of sex on the pharmacokinetic and pharmacodynamic properties of quinidine. British Journal of Clinical Pharmacology. 2003;**56**:198-204

[50] Ferrari M, Bolla E, Bortolaso P, Callegari C, Poloni N, Lecchini S, et al. Association between CYP1A2 polymorphisms and clozapine-induced adverse reactions in patients with schizophrenia. Psychiatry Research. 2012;**200**(2):1014-1017

[51] Franconi F, Campesi I. Pharmacogenomics, pharmacokinetics and pharmacodynamics: Interaction with biological differences between men and women. British Journal of Pharmacology. 2014;**171**(3):580-594

[52] Kearns GL, Abdel-Rahman SM, Alander SW, Blowey DL, Leeder JS, Kauffman RE. Developmental pharmacology–drug disposition, action, and therapy in infants and children. The New England Journal of Medicine. 2003;**349**:1157-1167

[53] Clavenna A, Bonati M. Adverse drug reactions in childhood: A review of prospective studies and safety alerts. Archives of Disease in Childhood. 2008;**94**:724-728

[54] Anderson GD, Lynn AM. AM. Optimizing pediatric dosing: A developmental pharmacologic approach. Pharmacotherapy. 2009;**29**(6):680-690

[55] Brown R, Dimond AR, Hulisz D, Saunders LA, Bobula JA. Pharmacoepidemiology of potential alcohol–prescription drug interactions among primary care patients with alcohol-use disorders. Journal of the American Pharmaceutical Association. 2007;**47**(2):135-139

[56] Coleman JJ, Ferner RE, McDowell SE. Systematic review and meta-analysis of ethnic differences in risks of adverse reactions to drugs used in cardiovascular medicine. BMJ. 2006;**332**:1177-1181

[57] Bruce R, Altice FL, Fried GH. Pharmacokinetic drug interactions between drugs of abuse and antiretroviral medications: Implications and management for clinical practice. Expert Review of Clinical Pharmacology. 2008;**1**(1):115-127

[58] Routledge P, O'mahony MS, Woodhouse KW. Adverse drug reactions in elderly patients. BJCP. 2003;**57**(2):121-126

[59] Prybys KM, Melville KA, Hanna JR, Gee PA. Polypharmacy in the elderly: Clinical challenges in emergency practice: Part I: Overview, etiology, and drug interactions. Emergency Medicine Reports. 2002;**23**(11):145-151

[60] Klotz U. Pharmacokinetics and drug metabolism in the elderly. Drug Metabolism Reviews. 2009;**41**(2):67-76

[61] Steinman MA, Seth Landefeld C, Rosenthal GE, Berthenthal D, Sen S, Kaboli J. Polypharmacy and precsribing quality in older people. Journal of the American Geriatrics Society. 2006;**54**(10):1516-1523

[62] Ahmed N, Mandel R, Fain MJ. Frailty: An emerging geriatric syndrome. The American Journal of Medicine. 2007;**120**(9):748-753

[63] Hilmer SN, McLachlan AJ, Le Couteur DG. Clinical pharmacology in the geriatric patient. Fundamental & Clinical Pharmacology. 2007;**21**(3):217-230

[64] Hutchison LC, O'Brien CE. Changes in pharmacokinetics and pharmacodynamics in the elderly patient. Journal of Pharmacy Practice. 2007;**20**(1):4-12

[65] Cannon KT, Choi MM, Zuniga MA. Potentially inappropriate medication use in elderly patients receiving home health care: A retrospective data analysis. The American Journal of Geriatric Pharmacotherapy. 2006;**4**(2):134-143

[66] Hajjar ER, Cafiero AC, Hanlon JT. Polypharmacy in elderly patients. The American Journal of Geriatric Pharmacotherapy. 2007;**5**:345-351

[67] Petrone K, Katz P. Approaches to appropriate drug prescribing for the older adult. Primary Care; Clinics in Office Practice. 2005;**32**:755-775

[68] American Geriatrics Society Clinical Practice Committee. The use of oral anticoagulants (warfarin) in older people. Journal of the American Geriatrics Society. 2002;**50**:1439

[69] Branch RA, James J, Read AE. A study of factors influencing drug disposition in chronic liver disease, using the model drug (+)-propranolol. British Journal of Clinical Pharmacology. 1976;**3**:243-249

[70] Dreisbach AW, Lertora JJ. The effect of chronic renal failure on hepatic drug metabolism and drug disposition. Seminars in Dialysis. 2003;**16**:45-50

[71] Frye RF, Zgheib NK, Matzke GR, Chaves-Gnecco D, Rabinovitz M, Shaikh OS, Branch RA. Liver disease selectively modulates cytochrome P450-mediated metabolism. Clinical Pharmacology and Therapeutics. 2006;**80**:235-245

[72] Hasselstrom J, Eriksson S, Persson A, Rane A, Svensson JO, Sawe J. The metabolism and bioavailability of morphine in patients with severe liver cirrhosis. British Journal of Clinical Pharmacology. 1990;**29**:289-297

[73] Ogasawara K, Terada T, Katsura T, Hatano E, Ikai I, Yamaoka Y, Inui K. Hepatitis C virus related cirrhosis is a major determinant of the expression levels of hepatic drug transporters. Drug Metabolism and Pharmacokinetics. 2010;**25**:190-199

[74] Sun H, Frassetto L, Benet LZ. Effects of renal failure on drug transport and metabolism. Pharmacology & Therapeutics. 2006;**109**(1-2):1-11

[75] Venitz R. Effect of chronic renal failure on the disposition of highly hepatically metabolized drugs. International Journal of Clinical Pharmacology and Therapeutics. 2000; **38**(5):245-253

[76] Yurdaguel Z, Christina C, Antje A, Eckhart GH, Harald D. Risk factors associated with adverse drug reactions following hospital admission: A prospective analysis of 907 patients in two German university hospitals. Drug Safety. 2008;**31**(9):789-798

[77] Macdonald JB, Macdonald B, Golitz LE, LoRusso P, Sekulic A. Cutaneous adverse effects of targeted therapies: Part I: Inhibitors of the cellular membrane. Journal of the American Academy of Dermatology. 2015;**72**(2):203-218

[78] Pack A, Davis AR, Kritzer J, Yoon A, Camus A. Antiepileptic drugs: Are women aware of interactions with oral contraceptives and potential teratogenicity. Epilepsy & Behavior. 2009;**14**(4):640-644

[79] Obreli-Neto PR, Nobili A, de Oliveira Baldoni A, Guidoni CM, de Lyra Júnior DP, Pilger D. Adverse drug reactions caused by drug–drug interactions in elderly outpatients: A prospective cohort study. European Journal of Clinical Pharmacology. 2012;**68**:1667-1676

[80] Pringle K, Ahern FM, Heller DA, Gold CH, Brown TV. Potential for alcohol and prescription drug interactions in older people. Journal of the American Geriatrics Society. 2005;**53**(11):1930-1936

[81] Schmiedl S, Rottenkolber M, Hasford J, Rottenkolber D, Farker K, Drewelow B, Thürmann P, et al. Self-medication with over-the-counter and prescribed drugs causing adverse-drug-reaction-related hospital admissions: Results of a prospective, long-term multi-Centre study. Drug Safety. 2014;**37**(4):225-235

[82] Brooks KM, George JM, Pau AK, Rupert A, Mehaffy C, De P, et al. Cytokine-mediated systemic adverse drug reactions in a drug-drug interaction study of Dolutegravir with once-weekly isoniazid and Rifapentine. Clinical Infectious Diseases. 2018

[83] Moore N, Pollack C, Butkerait P. Adverse drug reactions and drug–drug interactions with over-the-counter NSAIDs. Therapeutics and Clinical Risk Management. 2015;**11**: 1061-1065

[84] Aronson JK, editor. Meyler's Side Effects of Drugs: The International Encyclopedia of Adverse Drug Reactions and Interactions. Elsevier; 2015

Chapter 2

Pharmacokinetics and Disposition of Green Tea Catechins

Kai On Chu and Calvin C.P. Pang

Additional information is available at the end of the chapter

http://dx.doi.org/10.5772/intechopen.74190

Abstract

Green tea reportedly possesses many health beneficial effects as a beverage. Its usage has even been elevated to therapeutic level for treatment of diseases, including cancer, after increasing the catechin constituents in green tea extract or through purified catechins compounds. However, the therapeutic effectiveness of green tea extract or catechin formulae on different diseases is still questionable and inconsistent in reported studies. One reason is the low and variable bioavailability of catechins or unknown constituents in green tea extract. The plasma levels of total catechins are usually at submicromolar level which is well below the effective dose in many *in vitro* studies. Besides their variable chemical structures that cause heterogeneity of absorption, green tea catechins are subject to extensive metabolism by phase II process and catabolism by colonic microbes that result in complicated pharmacokinetics. It is essential to understand the factors affecting the pharmacokinetics and metabolic profiles in plasma and tissues based on animal and human studies before green tea catechins can be applied for therapeutic use.

Keywords: green tea extract, catechins, pharmacokinetics, bioavailability, absorption, metabolism

1. Introduction

Tea is the most commonly consumed beverage in most populations across the world. Leaves of the tea plant *Camellia sinensis* were processed by careful steaming and roasting to produce green tea for drinks. The major biologically active constituent of green tea is polyphenols, mainly catechins and their gallate derivatives: (+)-catechin (C), (−)-epicatechin (EC), (−)-gallocatechin (GC), (−)-epigallocatechin (EGC), (−)-catechin-3-gallate (CG), (−)-epicatechin-3-gallate (ECG), gallocatechin-3-gallate (GCG) and (−)-epigallocatechin-3-gallate (EGCG) (**Figure 1**).

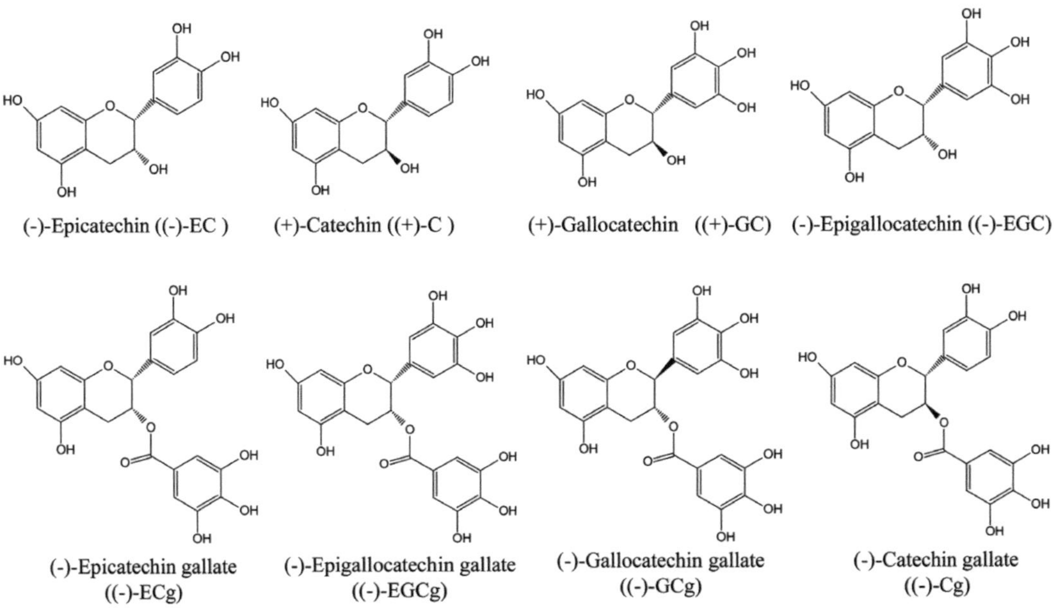

Figure 1. Structures of catechins.

Minor constituents include caffeine, theobromine, and theophylline. Among green tea catechins, EGCG is the most abundant and biologically active based on animal and human studies [1, 2]. The biological activity is attributed to its structure moiety and hydroxyl groups [3].

Health benefits are evident for green tea catechins including anticancer [4] and antimicrobial activities [5]. Cancer prevention has been found in the colon, duodenum, esophagus, stomach, large intestine, liver, lung, mammary glands, and skin [6, 7]. There were *in vitro* anticancer effects on adult T-cell leukemia (ATL) caused by a latent infection of human retrovirus HTLV-1 [8]. Drinking green tea could reduce HTLV-1 provirus load in asymptomatic HTLV-1 carriers [9]. Although the underlying mechanisms for cancer-prevention is not well understood, their antioxidation, free radical scavenger activities [10], and NF-κB inhibitory effect [11] have been attributed as the major factors.

Although biological and intervention studies have indicated various beneficial effects, results of clinical studies are not conclusive [12, 13]. Inconsistent findings may be attributed to variations of methodologies and study conditions such as differences in infusion techniques, consumption behavior, production methods, compositions of green tea constituents, and absorption profiles, among different study cohorts. Pharmacokinetics of green tea catechins have been studied using defined green tea catechin extract (GTE), Polyphenon E, and EGCG with variable doses of administration [14, 15]. Oral bioavailability of tea catechins in human plasma was found having 5 to 50 times lower than the level needed to exert biological activities in *in vitro* systems [16, 17]. Other studies showed very high free EGCG peak plasma concentrations, 300, 1970, and 2020 ng/mL, after ingestion of 3, 5, or 7 capsules of Sunphenon DCF-1 (containing 225, 375, and 525 mg EGCG), which is a green tea extract obtained by a defined protocol [18, 19]. Dosage affects the bioavailability of catechins. Many studies showed large variations of bioavailability of catechins which is related to their beneficial effects. Understanding the pharmacokinetics of catechins is important.

2. Pharmacokinetics of catechins

It is essential to know the effective concentrations and forms of catechins present in plasma and tissues after ingestion. Pharmacokinetics is a study of the absorption, distribution, metabolism, elimination, and bioavailability of catechins following administration. In brief, after oral administration of green tea or extract, catechins are absorbed from the small intestine and remaining excess catechins pass to the colon. In the small intestine, catechins are conjugated with glucuronic acid, sulfate or by O-methylation. Some catechins with secreted bile in an enterohepatic recirculation process pass into the colon and are degraded into different flavonoid rings by resident microorganisms. The catabolized phenolic acids can be reabsorbed into the circulation and excreted into urine. Catechins, their conjugated metabolites, and a large amount of catabolized small phenolic acids can be distributed to various organs and tissues, absorbed by tissue cells, further metabolized, and perform various biological actions (**Figure 2**).

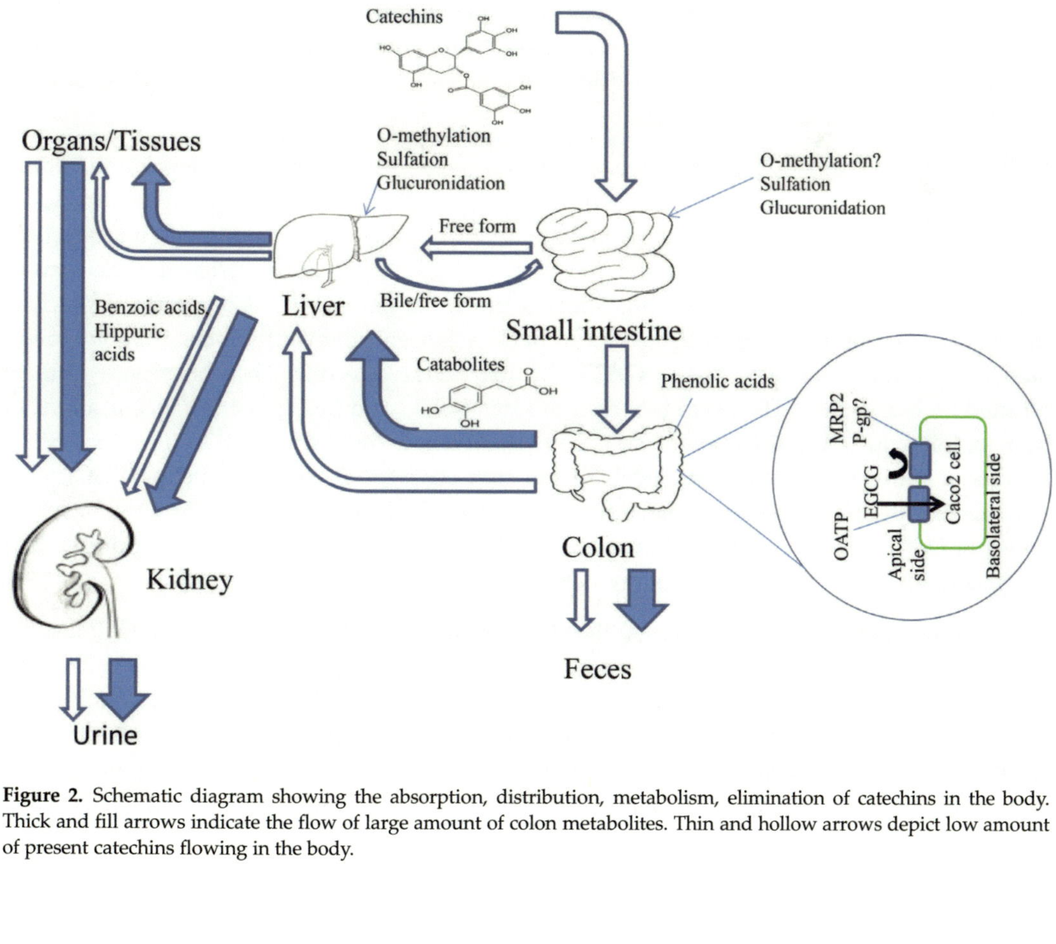

Figure 2. Schematic diagram showing the absorption, distribution, metabolism, elimination of catechins in the body. Thick and fill arrows indicate the flow of large amount of colon metabolites. Thin and hollow arrows depict low amount of present catechins flowing in the body.

3. Absorption

3.1. Conditions affecting absorption

Unlike other flavonoids, catechins exist as aglycone form. Their absorption is not influenced by glucosidase digestion in the small intestine [20]. They can be absorbed directly across the intestinal surface. The absorption depends on the physicochemical properties such as molecular size, steric configuration, solubility, hydrophilicity, pKa, and the presence of galloylated derivatives [21]. The presence of food matrix and drugs in the intestinal cavity also influences the absorption.

The oral bioavailability or catechins absorption is usually relatively low [22, 23]. The plasma concentration is usually 5–50 times less than the effective biological active concentrations in many *in vitro* studies [23]. In one study, green tea extract tablets containing 16.7 mg of EC, 44.9 mg of EGC, 11.1 mg of ECG, and 42.9 mg of EGCG were given to eight human subjects. Their mean maximum plasma levels (Cmax) were 34.7, 60.6, 20.9, and 42.8 ng/mL, respectively [24]. The absorption process of catechins and their metabolites may involve efflux transporters, like multidrug resistance-associated protein 2 (MRP2), in the small intestine resulting in low bioavailability [25]. It has been reported that ungallated catechins were effluxed by MRPs expressed in a Caco-2 monolayer cells model [26]. In human, a non-proportional surge of area under curve (AUC), Cmax, and total and free plasma level of EGCG appeared following increase of oral dosage of a green tea extract (GTE) preparation, Polyphenon E, from 800 to 1200 mg [27]. It was possible that the efflux mechanism was saturated at higher dose causing surge of catechins absorption at high dose.

P-glycoprotein (P-gp) is a transporter or efflux transporter for many molecules including catechins [28, 29]. EGCG can interact with P-gp and affect the absorption of other drugs. On the contrary, co-administration of some drugs can affect the absorption of green tea catechins [30]. Polymorphisms of P-gp in human and *in vitro* studies were associated with variations of Cmax and AUC of catechins after ingestion of green tea extract [31]. Competitive catechin-drug interaction of transporters also reduced plasma concentration of β-blocker nadolol mediated by organic anion-transporter OATP1A2 [32]. Oral catechins absorption can also be affected by food intake. The average maximum free EGCG and EGC plasma concentrations in human, following administration of the GTE Polyphenon E, increased 3.5-fold from the fasting condition. While the total plasma levels of free and conjugated epigallocatechin (EGC) were not affected, the plasma level of total epicatechins was lowered [33]. In addition, the bioavailability of EGCG taken in capsule form was 2.7 and 3.5 times higher from fasting condition than when taken with light breakfast or strawberry sorbet [34].

EGCG is stable in acidic condition as in the stomach but unstable in higher pH in the intestine. After passing through the stomach, the EGCG present in the gastric juice is neutralized by bicarbonate ions secreted by the pancreas in the duodenum where EGCG is degraded rapidly [29, 33]. Only about 1% EGCG can be measured in the small intestines after 1-h incubation [35]. Although the acidic condition in a strawberry sorbet or fruit juice could protect EGCG, the subsequently bicarbonate neutralization still leads to EGCG degradation. In addition, food can delay gastric emptying rate. The delay would subsequently reduce the Cmax (824.2 ± 75.1 ng/mL for EGCG without food; 231.8 ± 134.3 ng/mL and 218.0 ± 160.0 ng/mL with breakfast and strawberry sorbet) due to prolonging the time to Cmax (Tmax) (60 ± 34.6 min for EGCG without food; 120 ± 34.6 and 120 ± 34.6 min with breakfast and strawberry sorbet).

3.2. Absorption in the presence of food

On the other hand, lower bioavailability is not due to the elimination difference in the presence of food because the half-life of elimination was not significantly different between empty stomach and with food [36]. Moreover, food components could irreversibly and reversibly interact with catechins to affect their absorption in the proximal region of small intestine [37]. It also increased the viscosity of digestive fluid to reduce the dissolution of catechins [38], and induced bile acid secretion to promote elimination of the absorbed catechins. These are factors causing low oral and variable bioavailability of catechins. Despite catechins being stable in the stomach, the oligomer form of catechins, proanthocyanidins, are hydrolyzed to monomer or dimer in the acidic condition [39]. However, an *in vivo* study has not shown hydrolyzed product present in the gastric juice [36].

Milk has been reported to reduce catechin absorption [11] due to interaction with protein molecules [40]. Alcohol increased the solubility of catechins but did not increase plasma levels of catechins [41]. Co-administration of butter with tea, on the other hand, could decrease the Cmax of EGCG, EGC, EC, GCG, GC, and ECG by more than 40%. It also prolonged the mean residence times (MRT) of free EGCG, EGC, EC, GC and ECG by more than 40%. However, the levels of total (free and conjugated) catechins were not affected. Butter could modify catechins metabolism by increasing the conjugation in the intestine possibly through increasing the expression of UGT1A1 [42, 43]. Both forms of catechins excreted into feces increased from 124 to 232%. It suggests biliary secretion of EGCG, EGC, EC, GCG, and GC increased in response to lipid absorption. Similarly, obese SD rats with hyperlipidemia also increased fecal excretion of catechins from 0.52–1.3 to 1.2–3.4% when compared to normal rats. Lipids may alter the metabolism and the relative proportions of the microflora in the colon [44] and, subsequently, affect catechin catabolism. Since catechin catabolites have been attributed to many biological activities [45], the consequence of suppressing catechins metabolism remains to be elucidated. Furthermore, lipids can delay the gastric emptying causing Tmax increase [46]. Chocolate supplement caused the Tmax delay from 1–2 to 3.2–3.8 h [47].

In contrast to a lipid meal, carbohydrate rich meals, could increase the oral bioavailability (AUC) of flavanol by 140% [48]. The bioavailability of EGC and EGCG was significantly enhanced when administered with mixture of GTE (50 mg), sucrose and ascorbic acid (3237.0 and 181.8 pmol*h/L respectively) comparing to green tea (1304.1 and 61.0 pmol*h/L plasma respectively) in Sprague Dawley (SD) rats [49]. In addition, green tea mixed with vitamin C and xylitol also improved flavanols absorption in human. The Cmax, Tmax, and AUC of flavanols in plasma were 5980.58 μg/mL, 2.14 h, and 18,915.56 h.μg/mL, respectively comparing to the AUC of green tea control, 13,855.43 h.μg/mL. Sugar also delays gastric emptying, that in turns delays the Tmax [50]. Ascorbic acid and sucrose can improve catechin absorption through suppressing intestinal effluxing the absorbed catechins and stabilizing catechins in the lumen. Consistently, there was 6–11 times increase in intestinal uptake of total catechins comparing to green tea control following administered green tea with xylitol/citric acid and xylitol/vitamin C [51].

Besides the effect of food and drug interaction, we found catechins absorption steric and structural dependent [52]. In one study, we fed 550 mg/kg GTE to SD rats. After normalization with the input oral doses, the relative $AUC_{0\text{-}20\ h}$ of epi-isomers in the plasma was higher than its enantiomers, with the level of EGC > GC, EC > C, and EGCG>GCG. Also, the plasma levels of ungallated catechins (EGC, GC, and EC) were higher than gallated catechins (EGCG, GCG,

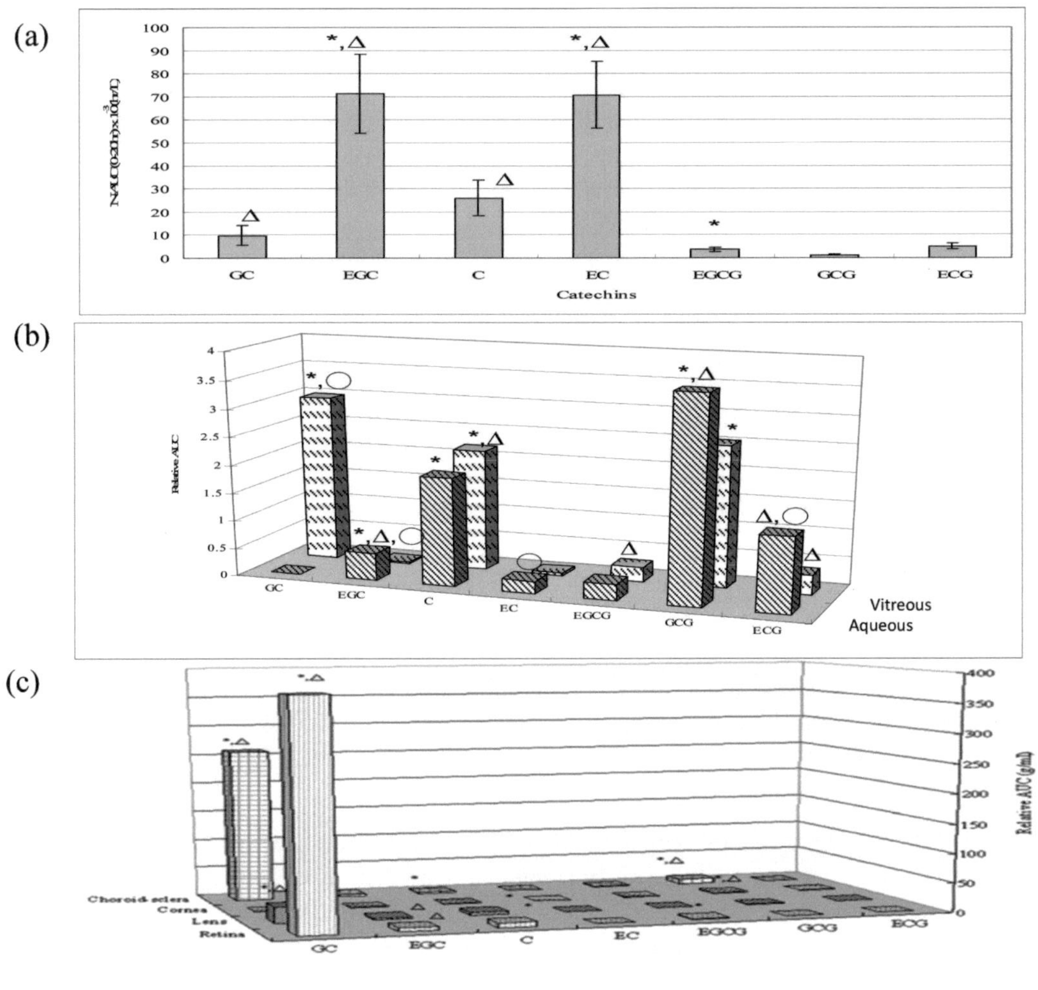

Figure 3. Diagrams showing the normalized relative AUC levels of total catechins (conjugated and free form) in ocular fluid and tissues. (a) Relative AUC levels of different catechins in the plasma after normalization by the corresponding input catechin dose in the GTE. Ungallate levels showed higher than gallate derivatives while epimers were higher than non-epimers. (b) Relative AUC levels of catechins in vitreous and aqueous humor. Vitreous humor showed selective to non-epimer but no selectivity on gallated and ungallated catechins. No particular trends of catechins selectivity appeared in aqueous humor. (c) Relative AUC levels of catechins in retina, lens, cornea and choroids-sclera. Adapted from Chu et al. [52].

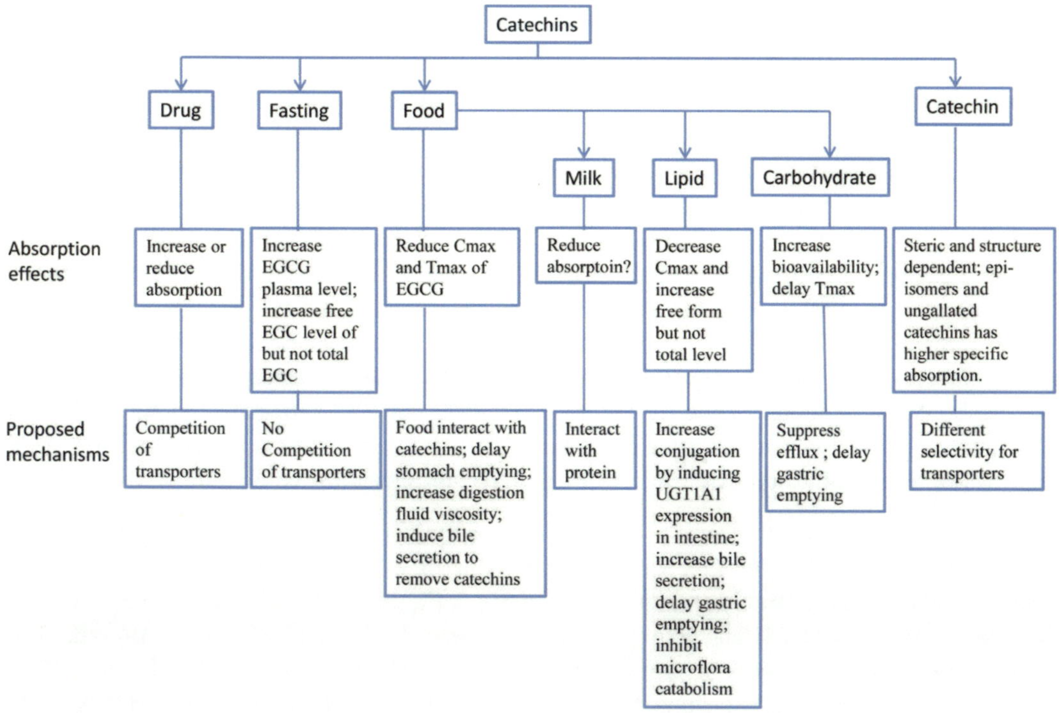

Figure 4. Summary of factors influencing the bioavailability and absorption.

and ECG) (**Figure 3**). Catechins absorption should involve selective mechanisms and different transporters. Moreover, when administrated with another GTE with higher proportion of EGCG orally, the relative AUC of GC is higher than EC while other patterns of the AUC levels remained the same [53]. It indicated that unknown interaction of absorptions between catechins and EGCG promotes catechin absorption. In addition, although EGCG is dominantly present in the GTE, its relative AUC level is very low, suggesting EGCG was not favorably absorbed in the intestine (**Figure 4**).

4. Metabolism

4.1. Effects of conjugations

Catechins are mainly metabolized by phase 2 conjugation processes through methylation, sulfation, and glucuronidation in the intestine and liver after oral administration. Glucuronidation and sulfation mainly occur in the intestine, whereas glucuronidation, sulfation, and methylation occur in the liver. Some conjugates are further methylated. Glucuronidation and sulfation can increase the polarity of catechins to enhance solubility and facilitate their eliminations through urine. EGCG, EGC and EC glucuronide and sulfate were commonly found in plasma [20, 27]. O-methyl-EGC-O-glucuronides and O-methyl-EC-O-sulfates were found in human urine [54] and methylated EGC conjugates were detected in human plasma after oral GTE administration [55], but the metabolites were not found in plasma in the other study [56].

A large amount of catechins were further catabolized by microflora in the colon, reabsorbed into plasma, and eliminated through urine. Major catechins catabolites were phenylvaleric acid and phenylvalerolactones, such as 5-(3′, 4′, 5′-trihydroxyphenyl)-γ-valerolactone (M4) and 5-(3′, 4′-dihydroxyphenyl)-γ-valerolactone (M6) [57]. They can be further metabolized and shortened to C6-C1 phenolic and aromatic acids, and then reabsorbed to enter the circulation and excreted into urine. These small phenolic acids can be conjugated to valerolactone-3′-O-sulfate, pyrogallol-2-O-sulfate, Pyrogallol-2-O-glucuronide, and vanilloylglycine for excretion in urine [58]. EGC and EC were metabolized into M4 and M6 and excreted likewise. EGCG was metabolized to EGC and 5-(3′,5′-dihydroxyphenyl)-γ-valerolactone in the rat. The amount of metabolites was about 6–39% of the ingested EGC and EC [59]. Elevated hippuric acid (N-benzoylglycine) in excretion after green tea consumption by healthy volunteers comparing to ileostomist also indicated extensive catabolism of catechins in the colon [60].

Owing to extensive metabolism, a wide variety of metabolites of catechins were found in the plasma and urine after green tea consumption [61]. Ten metabolites, in the form of O-methylated, sulfated, and glucuronide conjugates of EC and EGC, were identified in human plasma, where only low levels, 55 and 25 nM, of intact EGCG and ECG were present. The phase II catechin metabolites in urine were about 8% of the total catechin intake. Ileal fluid from ileostomist fed with catechins contained about 33% parent compounds and 37% of 23 catechins conjugates, similar to healthy subjects [62]. About 70% of the ingested catechins that were found as naïve catechins and conjugated metabolites, indicated that catechins were mainly metabolized after glucuronidation, sulfation and methylation, and were effluxed back into the lumen without extensive catabolism in the intestine. These compounds entered into the colon and were subsequently hydrolyzed by resident microflora to remove the conjugated moieties, releasing the aglycones and further catabolized into low molecular weight phenolic acids by ring fission. Consequently, substantial amount of the gallated catechins (47% of input dose) were detected in ileal fluid, and small amount of phenolic acids, pyrocatechol and pyrogallol derived from the gallic acid moiety, were detected in human urine after green tea consumption [63]. Other catabolites, 4-hydroxybenzoic acid, 5-(3,4,5-trihydroxyphenyl)-γ-valeric acid, 3-(3-hydroxyphenyl)-3-hydroxypropionic acid, hippuric acid, 3-methoxy-4-hydroxyphenylacetic acid, and 4-hydroxyphenylacetic acid, were also found in urine. These phenolic acid catabolites account to about 40% of the intake, and would account for the major biological activity of catechins instead of the low bioavailability of the parent compounds.

4.2. Microbial metabolism

The efficiency of microbial metabolism on catechins was well reported in a GTE study on cows [64]. Different doses of GTE was applied intraruminally (10 and 50 mg/kg) and duodenally (10, 20 and 30 mg/kg BW) to dairy cows. No catechin could be found in the plasma for both doses after intraruminal administration. However, plasma concentrations of EC, EGC, and EGCG were increased on increasing dosage after intraduodenal administration. It demonstrated the high metabolism efficiency of ruminal microorganisms under intraruminal administration.

4.3. Effects of metabolism on pharmacokinetics

Catechins are suffered from extensive and different types of metabolisms. Also, some conjugates formation, like sulfates, are resistant to enzymatic hydrolysis during the sample preparation of chemical analysis [65]. These are reasons contributing to the large variation of pharmacokinetics data in reported studies.

Catechins contain many epimers with different steric structures, the enantiomers are absorbed and metabolized differently. For example, absorption of (−)-C was lower than (+)-C [66]. A study on metabolism of flavan-3-ols in human males ingested with equal quantities of (−)-EC, (−)-C, (+)-EC, and (+)-C reported different bioavailability. The plasma and urine showed different levels of stereoisomers with (−)-EC > (+)-EC > (+)-C > (−)-C. Also, different levels of non-methylated conjugations, and 3′- and 4″-O-methylation of epimers were found, indicating stereoisomers can affect the metabolism of each other in the phase II metabolism [67]. Unlike ungallated catechin, the conjugation of gallate derivatives, such as ECG and EGCG, were not found in plasma and urine [68]. The galloyl moiety might inhibit phase II metabolism. In another study, about 50% of ingested EGCG was found from ileal fluid in ileostomists indicating EGCG was hardly absorbed. Only 1% of phase II conjugate of EGCG was detected in ileal fluid, showing excretion of EGCG directly from the enterocytes rather than being metabolized in the liver and entering into the enterohepatic recirculation [69].

5. Distribution

Most distribution studies were conducted in rodents. In one study, green tea polyphenols (0.6%) were given to rats for 8 days. Total (conjugated and free) EGC and EC levels were found in the bladder, large intestine, kidney, lung, and esophagus at 2–3, 1–3, 1–2, 0.5–1, 0.5–0.7 micromole levels, respectively. However, they were almost undetectable in spleen, liver, thyroid, and heart [70]. The total EGCG levels in large intestine, esophagus, and bladder were 1.1, 0.61, and 0.44 micromoles while kidney, prostate, spleen, liver, and lung were undetected. In a 12-day study in mice, Tmax of tea catechins in the lung and liver occurred on Day 4, but the level was decreased from then on. Catechin concentrations in the lung were always higher than that in the liver [67]. In an EGCG study on rats at 500 mg/kg orally, the Cmax of EGCG in the small intestine mucosa, colon mucosa, liver, plasma, and brain were 565, 69, 48, 12, and 0.5 μmol/L, respectively [68]. It appears the level of distribution is related to the extent of catechins contact to the tissues.

Furthermore, we found that catechins can be distributed into various ocular tissues including aqueous humor, vitreous humor, choroid-sclera, retina, lens, and cornea. After feeding 550 mg/kg GTE to SD rats, the Cmax of GC and ECG can reach to more than 10 and 1 μmol/kg, respectively, in the choroid-sclera and retina and 1 μmol/kg in the lens [52] (**Table 1**). Levels of catechins disposed in the ocular tissue could reach the effective dose. In our studies, green tea extract can exert anti-oxidation, anti-inflammation and anti-apoptotic effects on the ocular tissues especially for retina [52, 53, 69]. However, doubled the dose of EGCG in another GTE resulted surge of EGCG deposing in the ocular tissues and caused the retina turning to

	GC	EGC	C	EC	EGCG	GCG	ECG
Cmax (nM)							
Plasma	91.5 ± 57.4	754.9 ± 235.8	139.0 ± 57.0	1258.4 ± 294.0*	310.4 ± 59.9	50.8 ± 10.4	159.1 ± 33.9
Aqueous humor	–	602.9 ± 116.7*	127.4 ± 62.8	138.9 ± 58.5	13.2 ± 5.1	33.5 ± 20.4	47.8 ± 8.1
Vitreous humor	110.6 ± 22.1*	15.9 ± 7.0	96.5 ± 23.3*	20.5 ± 10.6	15.4 ± 2.7	20.9 ± 9.9	14.0 ± 5.1
Cmax (pmol/g)							
Choroid-sclera	11461.8 ± 5168.7*	1506.3 ± 941.1	477.6 ± 346.9	283.5 ± 66.5	184.4 ± 39.0	220.5 ± 69.7	10.7 ± 4.3
Retina	22729.4 ± 4229.4*	8020.8 ± 1658.49*	492.7 ± 235.2	608.0 ± 112.0	259.1 ± 67.2	3.2 ± 1.9	–
Lens	1558.1 ± 318.4*	1172.3 ± 207.8*	300.0 ± 151.5	72.3 ± 19.1	149.1 ± 26.5	18.0 ± 6.6	90.3 ± 45.8
Cornea	–	359.4 ± 66.8*	58.5 ± 15.4	30.6 ± 5.7	25.2 ± 15.5	10.7 ± 3.9	91.1 ± 18.7

Adapted from Chu et.al. [52].
* Indicates that the catechin(s) has significant higher ($p < 0.05$, $n = 6$) level of the parameter in the corresponding biological fluid or tissue than the others as analyzed by compared by nonparametric Kruskal-Wallis H method.

Table 1. Maximum concentration of catechins in plasma, humors, eye tissues after a single dose of 550 mg/kg of Sunphenon DCF-1 green tea extract administrated orally to rats.

pro-oxidative status and reducing the anti-apoptotic effect. Catechins disposition into ocular compartments also exhibited steric selectivity. Vitreous humor was selective to non-epimer catechins but without any structural preference to ungallated catechins as shown in the plasma. Ocular tissues, on the contrary, did not show any specific disposition except GC was dominated in retina, choroid-sclera, and the lens. Of note, it is our study on rat fetus. We also found catechins can penetrate into various fetal tissues, including brain, eye, lung, heart, liver, and kidney, following feeding to pregnant SD rat [71]. However, the Cmax levels of catechins were below micromolar level. The effective biological activity on the fetus is still questionable. Nevertheless, the Cmax of EGCG in the fetal eye could reach to 0.83 μM that may affect the ocular development in this critical stage.

We have found GTE, Theaphenon® E, containing 70% EGCG, exerted biological effects on various ocular diseases models. High oral dose of GTE, 550 mg/kg, suppressed various inflammation responses in the iris and ciliary body, and aqueous humor following LPS-induced ocular inflammation [69]. Our latest unpublished data also showed that it inhibited retina inflammation through reduction of microglial cells and suppression of astroglial reactions. In another sodium iodate-induced retina degeneration model, oral administration of 550 mg/kg Theaphenon® E or catechins mixtures containing 438 mg/kg EGCG could protect retina from disruptive folding caused by sodium iodate [72]. Such effects were possibly exerted through their anti-oxidative effects as demonstrated by the reduction of 8-iso-PGF2α, superoxide dismutase, and glutathione peroxidase levels in the retina. The anti-oxidative properties also contributed to cataract inhibition, through cataracto-static ability as convincingly revealed by Thiagarajan et al. [73]. The antioxidation protection was also supported by our previous study [53]. Theaphenon® E increased the GSH/GSSG ratio and reduced 8-iso-PGF2α level in the lens, although the catechins levels inside the lens was relative low comparing to other ocular tissues.

In a human study, green tea and black tea were given to patients 5 days prior to undergoing prostatectomy surgery. Four main catechins were found in the prostate tissue ranging from 21 to 107 pmol/g [74]. Similar amount of EGCG and 4″-O-methyl EGCG were found in the prostate tissue in a following study [75]. Since only trace amounts of 4″-O-methyl EGCG were present in human plasma after green tea consumption, it suggested that catechol O-methyltransferase was present in prostate to methylate EGCG [76].

6. Elimination

Catechins are mainly cleared through urinary and biliary excretion. Non-galloylated catechins are mainly excreted in urine in the form of parent and conjugated compounds. Galloylate catechins are mainly excreted through biliary excretion to the colon. In one study, minor epi- or gallocatechin-O-sulfates were detected in urine, while aglycones, ECG and EGCG, were absent after green tea consumption [68]. No conjugates of ECG and EGCG were detected in urine suggesting the gallate derivatives did not undergo phase II metabolism. The flavan-3-ol metabolites excreted were equivalent to 8.1% of ingested green tea flavan-3-ols [68]. Other studies found catechin metabolites accounted for 28.5% of intake, whereas gallocatechin metabolites accounted for 11.4% of the ingested (−)-epigallocatechin and (+)-gallocatechin [77]. EGCG cannot be detected in urine showing its elimination is not renal. On the other hand, EGCG may be degalloylated to other catechins in the liver after absorption through small intestine, subsequently metabolized and eliminated into urine resulting EGCG absent in there. However, EGCG and its metabolites could not be found in ileostomists urine suggested EGCG was not eliminated through the internal degalloylation process [78] because EGCG could be absorbed through colon and eliminated directly into urine. In addition, the half-lives of non-gallated catechins, EGC and EC, were shorter than gallated catechins, EGCG and ECg [31]. It may be because the more hydrophobic gallated catechins bind stronger to serum proteins and exist in non-conjugated free form that is not favorable for renal excretion [79, 80]. On the other hand, oral administration of catechins in rats found relative amounts of EC, EGCG, and ECG, respectively, at 4.72, 0.17, and 0.25% in urine and 11.0, 7.89, and 5.80% in feces [81]. In an isotope tracing study in rats, about 77% of the total radioactivity was present in bile but only 2.0% in the urine after intravenous administration of [4-^{3}H]-EGCG [82]. These evidences suggested that the galloyl catechin are excreted through the bile and eliminated through the feces.

In our study on GTE, Sunphenon, the elimination rates of catechins in retina and choroid-sclera were in general higher than the humors and plasma. The elimination rate was from 0.19 h^{-1} for GC to 2.4 h^{-1} in the retina, while the rate was from 0.04 for EGC to 0.24 for ECG in vitreous humor in SD rats [52]. However, when the dose of EGCG was doubled in another GTE, Theaphenon® E, we found the elimination rates of all catechins in the ocular tissues, particularly the retina, lower than the plasma [53] (**Table 2**). It appeared that some active elimination or metabolic mechanisms in ocular tissues facilitated the elimination. The elimination mechanism actively removed the catechins in the ocular tissues, but the mechanism was suppressed by the increased EGCG concentration. On the other hand, in our rat fetus study,

	GC	EGC	C	EC	EGCG	GCG	ECG
λz (h^{-1})							
(a)							
Plasma	0.107 ± 0.010	0.213 ± 0.015	0.104 ± 0.038	0.371 ± 0.000*	0.236 ± 0.007	0.171 ± 0.013	0.211 ± 0.010
Aqueous humor	–	0.045 ± 0.001	0.209 ± 0.012	0.093 ± 0.062	0.304 ± 0.012*	0.111 ± 0.033	0.124 ± 0.043
Vitreous humor	0.166 ± 0.010	0.041 ± 0.001	0.106 ± 0.030	0.067 ± 0.004	0.058 ± 0.012	0.042 ± 0.006	0.224 ± 0.035*
Choroid-sclera	0.057 ± 0.001	0.461 ± 0.015	0.220 ± 0.014	0.488 ± 0.007	0.267 ± 0.019	0.929 ± 0.049*	–
Retina	0.188 ± 0.045	0.203 ± 0.050	0.245 ± 0.010	2.432 ± 0.154*	0.413 ± 0.040	–	–
Lens	0.302 ± 0.049*	0.084 ± 0.020	0.234 ± 0.032	0.049 ± 0.004	0.269 ± 0.011	3.16 ± 0.13	–
Cornea	–	0.170 ± 0.031	0.116 ± 0.007	0.043 ± 0.012	0.125 ± 0.001	0.372 ± 0.006	0.477 ± 0.021*
(b)							
Plasma	0.27 ± 0.03	0.39 ± 0.04	0.37 ± 0.08	0.40 ± 0.05	0.23 ± 0.02	1.25 ± 0.38	0.21 ± 0.04
Aqueous humor	0.11 ± 0.02	0.24 ± 0.02	0.13 ± 0.03	0.21 ± 0.04	0.09 ± 0.02	–	0.13 ± 0.12
Vitreous humor	0.02 ± 0.01*	0.11 ± 0.09	0.11 ± 0.06	0.10 ± 0.03	0.08 ± 0.02	–	–
Choroid-sclera	–	0.25 ± 0.09	0.22 ± 0.09	0.37 ± 0.06	0.08 ± 0.04*	–	0.15 ± 0.07
Retina	–	0.04 ± 0.03	0.04 ± 0.01	0.06 ± 0.02	0.04 ± 0.02	–	0.09 ± 0.03
Lens	–	–	–	–	0.13 ± 0.06	–	–
Cornea	–	–	0.22 ± 0.10	0.22 ± 0.10	0.09 ± 0.02*	–	0.10 ± 0.09

Adapted from (a) Chu et al. [52] and (b) Chu et al. [53].
* Indicates that the catechin(s) has significant higher ($p < 0.05$, $n = 6$) level of the parameter in the corresponding biological fluid or tissue than the others as analyzed by compared by nonparametric Kruskal-Wallis H method.

Table 2. Elimination of catechins in plasma, humors, eye tissues after a single dose of 550 mg/kg of (a) Sunphenon DCF-1 green tea extract, and (b) Theaphenon® E administrated orally to rats.

the elimination rates of catechins in the maternal plasma, in general, were faster than the fetal tissues. The elimination rate of GC and EC were 0.26 and 0.3 h^{-1} for maternal plasma, whereas 0.08 and 0.1 h^{-1} for fetal kidney [71].

7. Conclusions

Many pharmacokinetics studies of green tea catechins were conducted on rodents and less studies in rabbits, dogs, or human. Most of them are oral administration studies. Although the plasma levels of total catechins are at submicromolar level, which is below the effective dose in many *in vitro* studies, tissue dispositions could be much higher. Ungallated catechins are mainly metabolized by phase II process in the small intestine and liver to form glucuronide/ sulfate conjugates in the plasma and urine while gallated catechins mostly remain intact in the plasma and are excreted through bile and metabolized by microflora in the colon. High levels of small metabolized phenolic acids can be reabsorbed into blood stream that may contribute to the *in vivo* biological effects.

Catechins can be widely distributed into various tissues including lung, eye, brain, gastrointestinal tract, kidney, bladder, and even passing through the placenta to the fetal organs. The disposition can be stereo-specific, and affected by food, drug, and catechins themselves indicating the absorption and distribution may involve some sort of transporters mechanisms. Before applying green tea catechins for therapeutic purpose, it is essential to understand their pharmacokinetics behavior and metabolites profiles not only in the plasma but also in various tissues in animals and in humans.

Author details

Kai On Chu and Calvin C.P. Pang*

*Address all correspondence to: cppang@cuhk.edu.hk

Department of Ophthalmology and Visual Sciences, The Chinese University of Hong Kong, Hong Kong

References

[1] Pastore RL, Fratellone P. Potential health benefits of green tea (Camellia sinensis): A narrative review. Explore (New York, NY). 2006;**2**:531-539. DOI: 10.1016/j.explore.2006.08.008

[2] Yang CS, Lambert JD, Ju J, Lu G, Sang S. Tea and cancer prevention: Molecular mechanisms and human relevance. Toxicology and Applied Pharmacology. 2007;**224**:265-273. DOI: 10.1016/j.taap.2006.11.024

[3] Du GJ, Zhang Z, Wen XD, Yu C, Calway T, Yuan CS, Wang CZ. Epigallocatechin Gallate (EGCG) is the most effective cancer chemopreventive polyphenol in green tea. Nutrients. 2012;**4**:1679-1691

[4] Butt MS, Ahmad RS, Sultan MT, Qayyum MM, Naz A. Green tea and anticancer perspectives: Updates from last decade. Critical Reviews in Food Science and Nutrition. 2015;**55**: 792-805. DOI: 10.1080/10408398.2012.680205

[5] Friedman M, Henika PR, Levin CE, Mandrell RE, Kozukue N. Antimicrobial activities of tea catechins and theaflavins and tea extracts against *Bacillus cereus*. Journal of Food Protection. 2006;**69**:354-361

[6] Serafini M, Ghiselli A, Ferro-Luzzi A. In vivo antioxidant effect of green and black tea in man. European Journal of Clinical Nutrition. 1996;**50**:28-32

[7] Dreosti IE, Wargovich MJ, Yang CS. Inhibition of carcinogenesis by tea: The evidence from experimental studies. Critical Reviews in Food Science and Nutrition. 1997;**37**:761-770. DOI: 10.1080/10408399709527801

[8] Li HC, Yashiki S, Sonoda J, Lou H, Ghosh SK, Byrnes JJ, Lema C, Fujiyoshi T, Karasuyama M, Sonoda S. Green tea polyphenols induce apoptosis in vitro in peripheral blood T lymphocytes of adult T-cell leukemia patients. Japanese Journal of Cancer Research. 2000;**91**:34-40

[9] Sonoda J, Koriyama C, Yamamoto S, Kozako T, Li HC, Lema C, Yashiki S, Fujiyoshi T, Yoshinaga M, Nagata Y, Akiba S, Takezaki T, Yamada K, Sonoda S. HTLV-1 provirus load in peripheral blood lymphocytes of HTLV-1 carriers is diminished by green tea drinking. Cancer Science. 2004;**95**:596-601

[10] Leung LK, Su Y, Chen R, Zhang Z, Huang Y, Chen ZY. Theaflavins in black tea and catechins in green tea are equally effective antioxidants. The Journal of Nutrition. 2001; **131**:2248-2251

[11] Gu JW, Makey KL, Tucker KB, Chinchar E, Mao X, Pei I, Thomas EY, Miele L. EGCG, a major green tea catechin suppresses breast tumor angiogenesis and growth via inhibiting the activation of HIF-1α and NFκB, and VEGF expression. Vascular Cell. 2013;**5**:9. DOI: 10.1186/2045-824X-5-9

[12] Zhong L, Goldberg MS, Gao YT, Hanley JA, Parent ME, Jin F. A population-based case-control study of lung cancer and green tea consumption among women living in Shanghai, China. Epidemiology. 2001;**12**:695-700

[13] Nagano J, Kono S, Preston DL, Mabuchi K. A prospective study of green tea consumption and cancer incidence, Hiroshima and Nagasaki (Japan). Cancer Causes & Control. 2001; **12**:501-508

[14] Chow HH, Cai Y, Alberts DS, Hakim I, Dorr R, Shahi F, Crowell JA, Yang CS, Hara Y. Phase I pharmacokinetic study of tea polyphenols following single-dose administration of epigallocatechin gallate and polyphenon E. Cancer Epidemiology, Biomarkers & Prevention. 2001;**10**:53-58

[15] Chow HH, Cai Y, Hakim IA, Crowell JA, Shahi F, Brooks CA, Dorr RT, Hara Y, Alberts DS. Pharmacokinetics and safety of green tea polyphenols after multiple-dose administration of epigallocatechin gallate and polyphenon E in healthy individuals. Clinical Cancer Research. 2003;**9**:3312-3319

[16] Hong J, Smith TJ, Ho CT, August DA, Yang CS. Effects of purified green and black tea polyphenols on cyclooxygenase- and lipoxygenase-dependent metabolism of arachidonic acid in human colon mucosa and colon tumor tissues. Biochemical Pharmacology. 2001; **62**:1175-1183

[17] Jung YD, Kim MS, Shin BA, Chay KO, Ahn BW, Liu W, Bucana CD, Gallick GE, Ellis LM. EGCG, a major component of green tea, inhibits tumour growth by inhibiting VEGF induction in human colon carcinoma cells. British Journal of Cancer. 2001;**84**:844-850. DOI: 10.1054/bjoc.2000.1691

[18] Nakagawa K, Okuda S, Miyazawa T. Dose-dependent incorporation of tea catechins, (−)-epigallocatechin-3-gallate and (−)-epigallocatechin, into human plasma. Bioscience, Biotechnology, and Biochemistry. 1997;**61**:1981-1985

[19] Yang CS, Chen L, Lee MJ, Balentine D, Kuo MC, Schantz SP. Blood and urine levels of tea catechins after ingestion of different amounts of green tea by human volunteers. Cancer Epidemiology, Biomarkers & Prevention. 1998;**7**:351-354

[20] Sesink AL, Arts IC, Faassen-Peters M, Hollman PC. Intestinal uptake of quercetin-3-glucoside in rats involves hydrolysis by lactase phlorizin hydrolase. The Journal of Nutrition. 2003;**133**:773-776

[21] Lee MJ, Wang ZY, Li H, Chen L, Sun Y, Gobbo S, Balentine DA, Yang CS. Analysis of plasma and urinary tea polyphenols in human subjects. Cancer Epidemiology, Biomarkers & Prevention. 1995;**4**:393-399

[22] Chen L, Lee MJ, Li H, Yang CS. Absorption, distribution, elimination of tea polyphenols in rats. Drug Metabolism and Disposition. 1997;**25**:1045-1050

[23] Lambert JD, Lee MJ, Lu H, Meng X, Hong JJ, Seril DN, Sturgill MG, Yang CS. Epigallocatechin-3-gallate is absorbed but extensively glucuronidated following oral administration to mice. The Journal of Nutrition. 2003;**133**:4172-4177

[24] Narumi K, Sonoda J, Shiotani K, Shigeru M, Shibata M, Kawachi A, Tomishige E, Sato K, Motoya T. Simultaneous detection of green tea catechins and gallic acid in human serum after ingestion of green tea tablets using ion-pair high-performance liquid chromatography with electrochemical detection. Journal of Chromatography. B, Analytical Technologies in the Biomedical and Life Sciences 2014;945–946:147-153. DOI: 10.1016/j.jchromb.2013.11.007

[25] Hong J, Lambert JD, Lee SH, Sinko PJ, Yang CS. Involvement of multidrug resistance-associated proteins in regulating cellular levels of (−)-epigallocatechin-3-gallate and its methyl metabolites. Biochemical and Biophysical Research Communications. 2003;**310**:222-227

[26] Zhang L, Zheng Y, Chow MS, Zuo Z. Investigation of intestinal absorption and disposition of green tea catechins by Caco-2 monolayer model. International Journal of Pharmaceutics. 2004;**287**:1-12. DOI: 10.1016/j.ijpharm.2004.08.020

[27] Chow HH, Hakim IA, Vining DR, Crowell JA, Ranger-Moore J, Chew WM, Celaya CA, Rodney SR, Hara Y, Alberts DS. Effects of dosing condition on the oral bioavailability of green tea catechins after single-dose administration of Polyphenon E in healthy individuals. Clinical Cancer Research. 2005;**11**:4627-4633. DOI: 10.1158/1078-0432.CCR-04-2549

[28] Song Q, Li D, Zhou Y, Yang J, Yang W, Zhou G, Wen J. Enhanced uptake and transport of (+)-catechin and (−)-epigallocatechin gallate in niosomal formulation by human intestinal Caco-2 cells. International Journal of Nanomedicine. 2014;**9**:2157-2165. DOI: 10.2147/IJN.S59331

[29] Spencer JP. Metabolism of tea flavonoids in the gastrointestinal tract. The Journal of Nutrition. 2003;**133**:3255S-3261S

[30] Jodoin J, Demeule M, Beliveau R. Inhibition of the multidrug resistance P-glycoprotein activity by green tea polyphenols. Biochimica et Biophysica Acta. 2002;**1542**:149-159

[31] Hung CC, Chiou MH, Teng YN, Hsieh YW, Huang CL, Lane HY. Functional impact of ABCB1 variants on interactions between P-glycoprotein and methadone. PLoS One. 2013; **8**:e59419. DOI: 10.1371/journal.pone.0059419

[32] Misaka S, Yatabe J, Müller F, Takano K, Kawabe K, Glaeser H, Yatabe MS, Onoue S, Werba JP, Watanabe H, Yamada S, Fromm MF, Kimura J. Green tea ingestion greatly reduces plasma concentrations of nadolol in healthy subjects. Clinical Pharmacology and Therapeutics. 2014;**95**:432-438. DOI: 10.1038/clpt.2013.241

[33] Spencer JP, Schroeter H, Rechner AR, Rice-Evans C. Bioavailability of flavan-3-ols and procyanidins: Gastrointestinal tract influences and their relevance to bioactive forms in vivo. Antioxidants & Redox Signaling. 2001;**3**:1023-1039. DOI: 10.1089/152308601317203558

[34] Naumovski N, Blades BL, Roach PD. Food inhibits the oral bioavailability of the major green tea antioxidant epigallocatechin gallate in humans. Antioxidants (Basel). 2015;**4**:373-393. DOI: 10.3390/antiox4020373

[35] Tenore GC, Campiglia P, Giannetti D, Novellino E. Simulated gastrointestinal digestion, intestinal permeation and plasma protein interaction of white, green, and black tea polyphenols. Food Chemistry. 2015;**169**:320-326. DOI: 10.1016/j.foodchem.2014.08.006

[36] Rios LY, Bennett RN, Lazarus SA, Rémésy C, Scalbert A, Williamson G. Cocoa procyanidins are stable during gastric transit in humans. The American Journal of Clinical Nutrition. 2002;**76**:1106-1110

[37] Welling PG. Effects of food on drug absorption. Annual Review of Nutrition. 1996;**16**:383-415. DOI: 10.1146/annurev.nu.16.070196.002123

[38] Reppas C, Eleftheriou G, Macheras P, Symillides M, Dressman JB. Effect of elevated viscosity in the upper gastrointestinal tract on drug absorption in dogs. European Journal of Pharmaceutical Sciences. 1998;**6**:131-139

[39] Spencer JP, Chaudry F, Pannala AS, Srai SK, Debnam E, Rice-Evans C. Decomposition of cocoa procyanidins in the gastric milieu. Biochemical and Biophysical Research Communications. 2000;**272**:236-241. DOI: 10.1006/bbrc.2000.2749

[40] Hollman PC, Van Het Hof KH, Tijburg LB, Katan MB. Addition of milk does not affect the absorption of flavonols from tea in man. Free Radical Research. 2001;**34**:297-300

[41] Donovan JL, Bell JR, Kasim-Karakas S, German JB, Walzem RL, Hansen RJ, Waterhouse AL. Catechin is present as metabolites in human plasma after consumption of red wine. The Journal of Nutrition. 1999;**129**:1662-1668

[42] Zhang L, Han Y, Xu L, Liang Y, Chen X, Li J, Wan X. The effects of co-administration of butter on the absorption, metabolism and excretion of catechins in rats after oral administration of tea polyphenols. Food & Function. 2015;**6**:2249-2256. DOI: 10.1039/c5fo00114e

[43] Osabe M, Sugatani J, Fukuyama T, Ikushiro S, Ikari A, Miwa M. Expression of hepatic UDP-glucuronosyltransferase 1A1 and 1A6 correlated with increased expression of the

nuclear constitutive androstane receptor and peroxisome proliferator-activated receptor alpha in male rats fed a high-fat and high-sucrose diet. Drug Metabolism and Disposition. 2008;**36**:294-302. DOI: 10.1124/dmd.107.017731

[44] Xu LW, Liang YH, Chen X, Chen B, Han YH, Zhang L. Hyperlipidemia affects the absorption, distribution and excretion of seven catechins in rats following oral administration of tea polyphenols. RSC Advances. 2015;**5**:97988-97994. DOI: 10.1039/C5RA19699J

[45] Chow HH, Hakim IA. Pharmacokinetic and chemoprevention studies on tea in humans. Pharmacological Research. 2011;**64**:105-112. DOI: 10.1016/j.phrs.2011.05.007

[46] Gentilcore D, Chaikomin R, Jones KL, Russo A, Feinle-Bisset C, Wishart JM, Rayner CK, Horowitz M. Effects of fat on gastric emptying of and the glycemic, insulin, and incretin responses to a carbohydrate meal in type 2 diabetes. The Journal of Clinical Endocrinology and Metabolism. 2006;**91**:2062-2067. DOI: 10.1210/jc.2005-2644

[47] Mullen W, Borges G, Donovan JL, Edwards CA, Serafini M, Lean MEJ, Crozier A. Milk decreases urinary excretion but not plasma pharmacokinetics of cocoa flavan-3-ol metabolites in humans. The American Journal of Clinical Nutrition. 2009;**89**:1784-1791. DOI: 10.3945/ajcn.2008.27339

[48] Schramm DD, Karim M, Schrader HR, Holt RR, Kirkpatrick NJ, Polagruto JA, Ensunsa JL, Schmitz HH, Keen CL. Food effects on the absorption and pharmacokinetics of cocoa flavanols. Life Sciences. 2003;**73**:857-869

[49] Peters CM, Green RJ, Janle EM, Ferruzzi MG. Formulation with ascorbic acid and sucrose modulates catechin bioavailability from green tea. Food Research International. 2010;**43**: 95-102. DOI: 10.1016/j.foodres.2009.08.016

[50] Phillips WT, Schwartz JG, Blumhardt R, McMahan CA. Linear gastric-emptying of hyperosmolar glucose solutions. Journal of Nuclear Medicine. 1991;**32**:377-381

[51] Shim SM, Yoo SH, Ra CS, Kim YK, Chung JO, Lee SJ. Digestive stability and absorption of green tea polyphenols: Influence of acid and xylitol addition. Food Research International. 2012;**45**:204-210. DOI: 10.1016/j.foodres.2011.10.016

[52] Chu KO, Chan KP, Wang CC, Chu CY, Li WY, Choy KW, Rogers MS, Pang CP. Green tea catechins and their oxidative protection in the rat eye. Journal of Agricultural and Food Chemistry. Feb 10, 2010;**58**:1523-1534. DOI: 10.1021/jf9032602

[53] Chu KO, Chan KP, Y2 Y, Qin YJ, Li WY, Chan SO, Wang CC, Pang CP. Effects of EGCG content in green tea extract on pharmacokinetics, oxidative status and expression of inflammatory and apoptotic genes in the rat ocular tissues. The Journal of Nutritional Biochemistry. 2015;**26**:1357-1367. DOI: 10.1016/j.jnutbio.2015.07.001

[54] Li C, Meng X, Winnik B, Lee MJ, Lu H, Sheng S, Buckley B, Yang CS. Analysis of urinary metabolites of tea catechins by liquid chromatography/electrospray ionization mass spectrometry. Chemical Research in Toxicology. 2001;**14**:702-707

[55] Meng X, Lee MJ, Li C, Sheng S, Zhu N, Sang S, Ho CT, Yang CS. Formation and identification of 4'-O-methyl-(−)-epigallocatechin in humans. Drug Metabolism and Disposition. 2001;**29**:789-793

[56] Wang JS, Luo H, Wang P, Tang L, Yu J, Huang T, Cox S, Gao W. Validation of green tea polyphenol biomarkers in a phase II human intervention trial. Food and Chemical Toxicology. 2008;**46**:232-240. DOI: 10.1016/j.fct.2007.08.007

[57] Li C, Lee MJ, Sheng S, Meng X, Prabhu S, Winnik B, Huang B, Chung JY, Yan S, Ho CT, et al. Structural identification of two metabolites of catechins and their kinetics in human urine and blood after tea ingestion. Chemical Research in Toxicology. 2000;**13**:177-184

[58] van der Hooft JJJ, de Vos RCH, Mihaleva V, Bino RJ, Ridder L, de Roos N, Jacobs DM, van Duynhoven J, Vervoort J. Structural elucidation and quantification of phenolic conjugates present in human urine after tea intake. Analytical Chemistry. 2012;**84**:7263-7271. DOI: 10.1021/ac3017339

[59] Kohri T, Matsumoto N, Yamakawa M, Suzuki M, Nanjo F, Hara Y, Oku N. Metabolic fate of (−)-[4-(3)H]epigallocatechin gallate in rats after oral administration. Journal of Agricultural & Food Chemistry. 2001;**49**:4102-4112. DOI: 10.1021/jf001491+

[60] Mulder TP, Rietveld AG, van Amelsvoort JM. Consumption of both black tea and green tea results in an increase in the excretion of hippuric acid into urine. The American Journal of Clinical Nutrition. 2005;**81**(Suppl):256S-260S

[61] Stalmach A, Troufflard S, Serafini M, Crozier A. Absorption, metabolism and excretion of Choladi green tea flavan-3-ols by humans. Molecular Nutrition & Food Research. 2009;**53** (Suppl 1):S44-S53. DOI: 10.1002/mnfr.200800169

[62] Stalmach A, Mullen W, Steiling H, Williamson G, Lean ME, Crozier A. Absorption, metabolism, and excretion of green tea flavan-3-ols in humans with an ileostomy. Molecular Nutrition & Food Research. 2010;**54**:323-334. DOI: 10.1002/mnfr.200900194

[63] Roowi S, Stalmach A, Mullen W, Lean ME, Edwards CA, Crozier A. Green tea flavan-3-ols: Colonic degradation and urinary excretion of catabolites by humans. Journal of Agricultural and Food Chemistry. 2010;**58**:1296-1304. DOI: 10.1021/jf9032975

[64] Wein S, Beyer B, Gohlke A, Blank R, Metges CC, Wolffram S. Systemic absorption of catechins after intraruminal or intraduodenal application of a green tea extract in cows. PLoS One. 2016;**11**:e0159428. DOI: 10.1371/journal.pone.0159428

[65] Saha S, Hollands W, Needs PW, Ostertag LM, de Roos B, Duthie GG, Kroon PA. Human O-sulfated metabolites of (2)-epicatechin and methyl-(2)-epicatechin are poor substrates for commercial aryl-sulfatases: Implications for studies concerned with quantifying epicatechin bioavailability. Pharmacological Research. 2012;**65**:592-602. DOI: 10.1016/j.phrs.2012.02.005

[66] Donovan JL, Crespy V, Oliveira M, Cooper KA, Gibson BB, Williamson G. (+)-Catechin is more bioavailable then (−)-catechin: Relevance to the bioavailability of catechin from cocoa. Free Radical Research. 2006;**40**:1029-1034. DOI: 10.1080/10715760600868545

[67] Ottaviani JI, Momma TY, Heiss C, Kwik-Uribe C, Schroeter H, Keen CL. The sterochemical configuration of flavanols influences the level and metabolism of flavanols in humans and their biological activity in vivo. Free Radical Biology & Medicine. 2011;**50**: 237-244. DOI: 10.1016/j.freeradbiomed.2010.11.005

[68] Nakagawa K, Miyazawa T. Absorption and distribution of tea catechin, (−)-epigallo-catechin-3- gallate, in the rat. Journal of Nutritional Science & Vitaminology. 1997;**43**:679-684

[69] Qin YJ, Chu KO, Yip YW, Li WY, Yang YP, Chan KP, Ren JL, Chan SO, Pang CP. Green tea extract treatment alleviates ocular inflammation in a rat model of endotoxin-induced uveitis. PLoS One. 2014;**9**:e103995. DOI: 10.1371/journal.pone.0103995

[70] Kim S, Lee MJ, Hong J, Li C, Smith TJ, Yang GY, Seril DN, Yang CS. Plasma and tissue levels of tea catechins in rats and mice during chronic consumption of green tea polyphenols. Nutrition & Cancer. 2000;**37**:41-48. DOI: 10.1207/S15327914NC3701_5

[71] Chu KO, Wang CC, Chu CY, Choy KW, Pang CP, Rogers MS. Uptake and distribution of catechins in fetal organs following in utero exposure in rats. Human Reproduction. 2007; **22**:280-287. DOI: 10.1093/humrep/del353

[72] Yang YP, Qin YJ, Yolanda Yip WY, Chan KP, Chu KO, Chu WK, Ng TK, Pang CP, Chan SO. Green tea catechins are potent anti-oxidants that ameliorate sodium iodate-induced retinal degeneration in rats. Scientific Reports. 2016;**6**:29546. DOI: 10.1038/srep29546

[73] Thiagarajan G, Chandani S, Sundari CS, Rao SH, Kulkarni AV, Balasubramanian D. Antioxidant properties of green and black tea, and their potential ability to retard the progression of eye lens cataract. Experimental Eye Research. 2001 Sep;**73**(3):393-401. DOI: 10.1006/exer.2001.1049

[74] Henning SM, Aronson W, Niu Y, Conde F, Lee NH, Seeram NP, Lee RP, Lu J, Harris DM, Moro A, et al. Tea polyphenols and theaflavins are present in prostate tissue of humans and mice after green and black tea consumption. The Journal of Nutrition. 2006;**136**:1839-1843

[75] Wang P, Aronson WJ, Huang M, Zhang Y, Lee RP, Heber D, Henning SM. Green tea polyphenols and metabolites in prostatectomy tissue: Implications for cancer prevention. Cancer Prevention Research (Philadelphia, PA). 2010;**3**:985-993. DOI: 10.1158/1940-6207. CAPR-09-0210

[76] Meng X, Sang S, Zhu N, Lu H, Sheng S, Lee MJ, Ho CT, Yang CS. Identification and characterization of methylated and ring-fission metabolites of tea catechins formed in humans, mice, and rats. Chemical Research in Toxicology. 2002;**15**:1042-1050

[77] Manach C, Williamson G, Morand C, Scalbert A. Re'me'sy C. Bioavailability and bioefficacy of polyphenols in humans. I. Review of 97 bioavailability studies. The American Journal of Clinical Nutrition. 2005;**81**:230S-242S

[78] Auger C, Hara Y, Crozier A. Bioavailability of polyphenon E flavan-3-ols in humans with an ileostomy. The Journal of Nutrition. 2008;**138**(Suppl):1535S-1542S

[79] Ishii T, Ichikawa T, Minoda K, Kusaka K, Ito S, Suzuki Y, Akagawa M, Mochizuki K, Goda T, Nakayama T. Human serum albumin as an antioxidant in the oxidation of (−)-epigallocatechin gallate: Participation of reversible covalent binding for interaction and stabilization. Bioscience, Biotechnology, and Biochemistry. 2011;**75**:100-106. DOI: 10.1271/bbb.100600

[80] Ishii T, Minoda K, Bae MJ, Mori T, Uekusa Y, Ichikawa T, Aihara Y, Furuta T, Wakimoto T, Kan T, Nakayama T. Binding affinity of tea catechins for HSA: Characterization by high-performance affinity chromatography with immobilized albumin column. Molecular Nutrition & Food Research. 2010;**54**:816-822. DOI: 10.1002/mnfr.200900071

[81] Zhu M, Chen Y, Li RC. Oral absorption and bioavailability of tea catechins. Planta Medica. 2000;**66**:444. DOI: 10.1055/s-2000-8599

[82] Kohri T et al. Synthesis of (−)-[4-3H]epigallocatechin gallate and its metabolic fate in rats after intravenous administration. Journal of Agricultural and Food Chemistry. 2001;**49**: 1042. DOI: 10.1021/jf0011236

Chapter 3

A Critical Risk Factor for a Major Side Effect of Interferon-Alpha Therapy: Activated Indoleamine 2,3-Dioxygenase 1 is Related to Depressive Symptoms

Yuki Murakami and Yukio Imamura

Additional information is available at the end of the chapter

http://dx.doi.org/10.5772/intechopen.71013

Abstract

Hepatitis C virus (HCV) infection affects approximately 170 million people worldwide. Interferon-alpha (IFN-α) is a cytokine that is related to early viral infection and has both antiviral and antiproliferative properties. The current standard treatment for long-term chronic hepatitis C (CHC) consists of combination therapy with IFN-α and ribavirin, which has a broad spectrum antiviral effect. Despite the potential therapeutic benefits of IFN-α, its administration often causes many side effects, such as somatic and neuropsychiatric symptoms. Depression is a serious and frequently occurring side effect of IFN-α therapy, and this is one of the major reasons for cessation of the therapy. Therefore, in order to avoid the discontinuation of INF-α therapy owing to depressive symptoms, it is important to identify the risk factor(s) leading to the onset of associated depressive symptoms. In this chapter, we introduce our novel findings on the association between IFN treatment and the onset of depression in CHC patients as well as the potential neurobiological mechanisms by which depression may arise. We also highlight a potential approach for predicting the onset risk of depression as a side effect in these patients.

Keywords: hepatitis C, IFNs, depression, tryptophan catabolism, indoleamine 2,3-dioxygenase 1

1. Introduction

Hepatitis C virus (HCV) infection is a global health problem. Up to 85% of HCV-infected patients may develop long-term chronic hepatitis C (CHC), a disease state associated with serious clinical sequela, including liver cirrhosis, hepatic fibrosis, and hepatocellular carcinoma [1–4]. It has been estimated that up to 20% of CHC patients will develop hepatic cirrhosis over a 20–25-year period, and these individuals are at an increased risk for developing end-stage hepatic diseases or hepatocellular carcinoma [4]. Therefore, aggressive antiviral treatments to successfully induce viral remission constitute a major strategy for reducing the morbidity and mortality associated with CHC.

Immunotherapy with interferon-alpha (IFN-α) is commonly used to treat CHC and several types of malignancies owing to its antiviral, antiproliferative, and immunoregulatory effects [5]. In clinical trials, more than 50% of CHC patients treated with combination therapy using IFN-α and ribavirin achieved a sustained viral response, defined as undetectable HCV in the blood 6 months following the end of treatment [4]. Despite the efficacy of IFN-α in CHC treatment, IFN-α therapy causes serious side effects; early signs include somatic symptoms (anorexia, pain, insomnia, fever, and fatigue). Prolonged therapy causes neuropsychiatric symptoms including depressive states, anhedonia, anxiety, and cognitive impairment. In particular, depression is a serious and frequently occurring side effect of IFN-α therapy, and this leads to discontinuation of the therapy in up to 45% of patients [6, 7]. Therefore, in order to avoid the discontinuation of IFN-α therapy owing to depressive symptoms induced by the cytokine, it is important to identify the risk factor(s) leading to the associated depressive symptoms.

A number of findings suggest that the neuropsychiatric side effects observed during IFN-α therapy may be linked to aberrations in the tryptophan (TRP)-kynurenine (KYN) pathway [8, 9]. Clinical studies have found that IFN-α therapy reduces plasma TRP and serotonin (5-hydroxythrptamine; 5-HT) levels [8] and increases KYN levels in plasma and cerebrospinal fluid (CSF). In addition, the KYN/TRP ratio, an index of indoleamine 2,3-dioxygenase 1 (IDO1) activity, is increased in patients receiving IFN-α therapy [8].

IDO1 is an extrahepatic enzyme that catalyzes the conversion of TRP to KYN, which can produce many neuroactive metabolites such as 3-hydroxykynurenine (3-HK), kynurenic acid (KA), and quinolinic acid (QUIN). Intriguingly, QUIN levels in CSF have been found to correlate with the severity of depressive pathology [10], and post-mortem studies have shown increased microglia QUIN levels in the frontal cortex of severely depressed patients [11].

In the current chapter, we present the findings of our latest study, which demonstrates the association between IFN treatment and changes in the TRP-KYN pathway in the blood of HCV patients. To do so, we investigated the effect of chronic *Ifn* gene expression on depression-like behavior and levels of brain TRP-KYN metabolites in mice. Our results suggest the possibility for the prediction of onset risk of depression as a side effect in HCV patients.

2. Molecular characteristics and antiviral mechanisms of interferons (IFNs)

2.1. Classification of IFNs

IFNs were first introduced in 1957 as antiviral molecules. Based on their receptor types on the cell membrane surface, IFNs are classified into type I and type II. IFN type I mainly consists of IFN-α/β, while IFN type II consists of IFN-γ. IFN type I is a family of cytokines in which their amino acid sequence similarity reaches 30–80%. They are produced by a wide variety of cells, including fibroblasts, epithelial cells, and hepatocytes [12, 13]. However, in most viral infections, plasmacytoid dendritic cells (pDCs) are probably the major source of these cytokines. In contrast, IFN type II (IFN-γ) is a single gene cytokine unrelated in structure to IFN-α/β, which is produced largely by macrophages, natural killer (NK) cells, and T lymphocytes [12].

2.2. Immune response for HCV infection and IFN induction

The host response against HCV infection is first triggered when a pathogen-associated molecular pattern (PAMP), presented by an infecting virus, is recognized and engaged by specific PAMP receptors expressed on the host cells. This leads to the activation of signals that ultimately induce the expression of antiviral effector genes [14, 15] (**Figure 1**). For RNA viruses, protein, and nucleic acid products of infection or replication have been identified as viral PAMPs. These are engaged by specific toll-like receptors (TLRs) or nucleic acid-binding proteins that serve as PAMP receptors [15–17]. The viral RNA of HCV contains each of these PAMP signatures, and is adequate to trigger the host response when introduced into naïve cells [18, 19]. In hepatocytes, which is the target cell of HCV infection, independent pathways

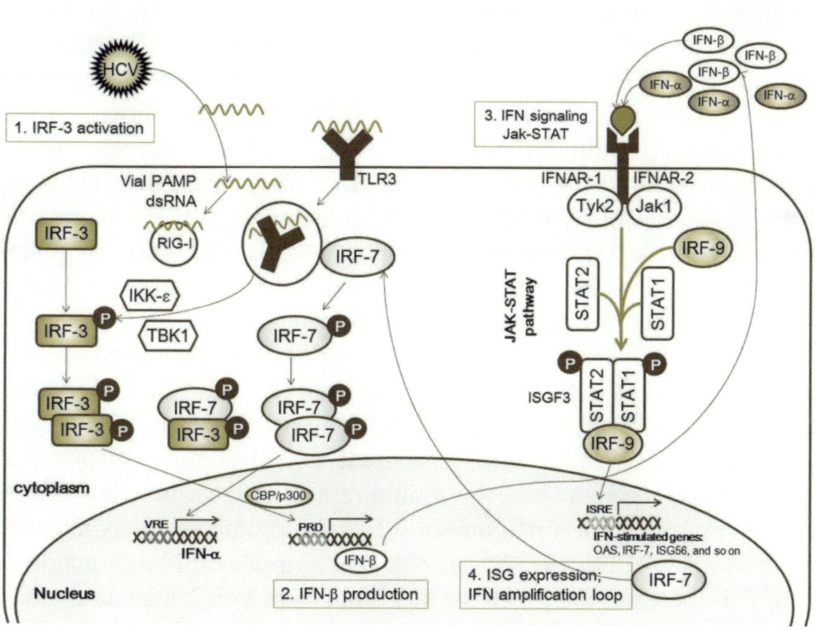

Figure 1. The host innate response to HCV infection. Adapted from Ref. [14]. (1) HCV RNA binding to RIG-I or TLR3 results in the activation IRF-3. The dimer of phospho-IRF-3 translocates to the nucleus, interacts with transcription partners and binds to the cognate-DNA PRD in the promoter region of IRF-3 target genes. (2) IRF-3 activation leads to the induction of IFN-β production. (3) Secreted IFN-β from the infected cells binds to the IFN-α/β receptor, and results in activation of the JAK-STAT pathway. The ISGF3 complex translocates to the nucleus, where it binds to the ISRE on target genes to direct ISG expression. IRF-7 is one of the ISGs and it is activated after expression through viral PAMP signaling. (4) The IRF-7 dimer and heterodimer with IRF-3 binds to VRE in the promotor region of IFN-α genes resulting in the production of various IFN-α subtypes and establishing a positive-feedback loop for IFN amplification. It is the IFN-α component of the host response that is exploited by the current IFN-based therapy for HCV infection [14].

of retinoic acid-inducible gene I (RIG-I) and TLR3 signaling construct two major pathways of host defense triggered by double-stranded (ds) RNA [19–21]. Viral PAMP binding to RIG-I or TLR3 results in the phosphorylation and activation of interferon regulatory factor 3 (IRF-3) by TANK-binding kinase 1 (TBK-1) and I kappa B kinase ε (IKK-ε) [14, 22]. The dimer of phospho-IRF-3 translocates to the cell nucleus, interacts with its transcription partners, including CREB-binding protein (CBP)/p300, and binds to the cognate-DNA positive regulatory domain (PRD) in the promoter region of IRF-3 target genes, such as IFN-β [14, 23]. The engagement of PAMP receptors also leads to the synthesis of IFN-α/β, tumor necrosis factor (TNF), and a variety of other cytokines, which are largely produced by mainly pDCs that express TLRs in abundance. IFN-α/β produced by pDCs activates NK cells, thereby enhancing their cytotoxic potential and stimulating their production of IFN-γ. IFN-α/β produced by pDCs also modulates the activation of $CD8^+$ T cells, which produce additional IFN-γ and represent the central players in the pathogen-specific adaptive immune response [12].

2.3. The antiviral effect of IFNs on HCV

IFN-α mediates a wide range of biological activities including antiproliferation, immunomodulation, and antiviral responses. IFN-α/β acts to induce the antiviral response in cells. These cells can be far from IFN-α/β production site and IFN-α/β interacts with specific cell surface receptors, type I IFN receptors (interferon-alpha receptor 1 (IFNAR1) and IFNAR2; **Figure 1**). IFNARs signal to the nucleus via Janus kinase-1 (Jak1) and tyrosine kinase 2 (Tyk2) phosphorylation of the signal transducers and activators of transcription (STATs) [24]. The classic IFN-α/β signaling pathways activate STAT1/STAT2 heterodimers and the trimeric IFN-stimulated gene factor (ISGF) complex containing IRF-9, which activate the expression of specific subsets of genes controlled by promoters containing interferon-stimulated response elements (ISRE; **Figure 1**) [15]. Interferon-stimulated genes (ISGs) are the genetic effectors of the host response, although the details of the signaling mechanisms by which IFN-α/β and IFN-γ induce the transcription of ISGs are still being defined [25]. IRF-7 is a transcription factor and an ISG. It is expressed in many tissue types, including complex liver tissue, in response to IFN. IRF-7 is activated after expression via viral PAMP signaling pathways that overlie with the IRF-3 activation pathway. IRF-7 phosphorylation, dimerization, and heterodimerization with IRF-3 lead to bind its cognate virus-responsive element (VRE) in the promotor region of IFN-α genes. Then, this binding results in the production of various IFN-α subtypes. The transcription effector action of IRF-7 also promotes diversification of the ISG response, establishing a positive-feedback loop that amplifies IFN production, and antiviral action [14]. This increases the plenty of RIG-I and viral PAMP signaling modules whose continued signaling acts to amplify IFN production and the host response. The medicinal administration of IFN-α promotes an antiviral reaction against HCV infection by stimulating ISG expression via the IFN-α/β receptor and the JAK-STAT pathway. In addition to stimulating ISG expression, IFN-α induces or promotes the maturation of immune effector cells, and enhances the production of other cytokines by resident hepatic cells to indirectly modulate the cell-mediated defenses and adaptive immunity to HCV [15]. Viral trigger and control of the host response may elucidate cellular tolerance for HCV RNA replication and influence the outcome of infection.

http://dx.doi.org/10.5772/intechopen.71013

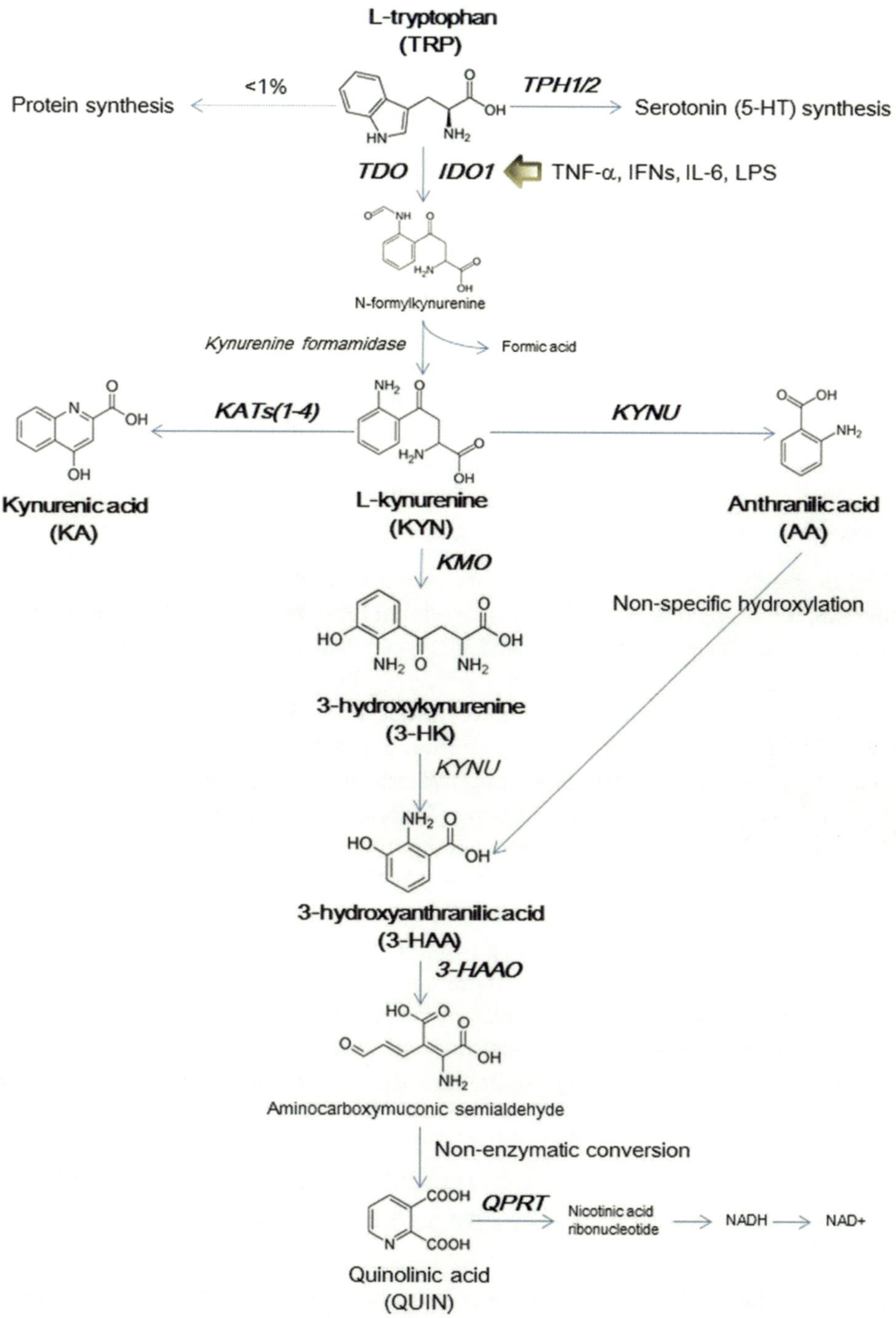

Figure 2. Schematic overview of the TRP-KYN pathway. IDO1 catabolizes L-TRP to N-formyl-L-kynurenine, which is converted to L-KYN by formamidase. L-KYN is further metabolized to AA by kynureninase (KYNU), to KA by kynurenine aminotransferases (KATs), and to 3-HK by kynurenine 3-monooxygenase (KMO). KMO is then metabolized to 3-HAA by 3-hydroxyanhranilate 3,4-dioxygenase (3-HAAO). 3-HAA is further metabolized to QUIN.

3. Side effect: IFN-induced depression and tryptophan metabolism

IFN-α has been shown to develop depression in many diseases, not only CHC, but also in melanoma, chronic myelogenous leukemia, and renal cell carcinoma [26]. However, CHC patients may be more susceptible to developing IFN-induced depression than patients with other disorders, possibly due to a baseline 5-HT system dysfunction. Depression in CHC patients may result from changes in platelet 5-HT function, with decreased 5-HT concentrations during CHC infection compensated for by a decrease in reuptake and metabolism [1]. Immune activation, particularly by IFN-γ, affects the catabolism of TRP, a precursor of 5-HT, by inducing expression of IDO1. IDO1 is the first and rate-limiting enzyme that converts TRP to N-formyl-L-kynurenine, which is further metabolized to QUIN (**Figure 2**). IFN treatment of CHC patients results in a decrease in plasma TRP and an increase in plasma KYN [8]. Another clinical study with cancer patients has shown that immunotherapy with IFN-α significantly increases the severity of depressive symptoms, which is related to a depletion of serum 5-HT and induction of the catabolism of TRP to KYN [27]. Thus, TRP catabolism switches from the 5-HT pathway to the KYN pathway, resulting in a decrease in 5-HT levels.

IDO1 is induced by several pro-inflammatory cytokines including IFNs (IFN-α/β, γ), TNF-α, and interleukin 6 (IL-6). It is also widely accepted that IFNs, especially IFN-γ, are essential factors for IDO1 induction since two ISREs and IFN-γ-activated site (GAS) element sequences are found in the 5′-flanking region of the IDO1 gene [28]. Recent preclinical studies in mice have demonstrated that pharmacological inhibition of IDO1 enzymatic activity or genetic deletion of IDO1 abrogates acute and chronic inflammation-dependent behavioral changes induced by peripheral or central administration of lipopolysaccharide (LPS) [29–33]. Additionally, it has been reported that peripheral administration of KYN alone can induce depression-like behavior in rats [34]. In a clinical study, patients receiving IFN-α therapy showed increases in the total Montgomery-Asberg Depression Rating Score (MADRS), an index of depressive symptoms similar to the KYN/TRP ratio; this indicates IDO1 activity and the KYN/KA ratio, which reflects a neurotoxic challenge [35]. These findings suggest that only TRP depletion itself may not be required for the induction of behavioral changes as a result of IDO1 activation; and that KYN and its neuroactive metabolites are more related to cytokine-induced depression-like behaviors than TRP depletion. However, it is still unclear whether direct activation of IDO1 and KYN metabolites plays a definitive role in the induction of depressive symptoms by IFN-α treatment.

4. The association between IFN treatment and changes in the TRP-KYN pathway on depression as a side effect in humans and mice

4.1. Changes in the levels of serum TRP and its metabolites in HCV patients with IFN-α therapy

In order to further clarify the relationship between the IDO1-induced KYN pathway and the development of depressive symptoms during IFN-α therapy, we conducted a study in which we measured TRP metabolites of the KYN pathway in the serum of HCV patients undergoing IFN-α therapy.

A total of 49 patients (32 males and 17 females; mean age 54.0 ± 2.3 years) suffering from CHC were recruited. **Table 1** shows the clinical characteristics of patients with HCV. In this study, most of patients were treated with recombinant (r) IFN-α 2b or pegylated (PEG)-IFN-α 2b (21 patients (42.9%) received each medicine, respectively). Five patients (10.2%) were treated with natural (n) IFN-α, and others received PEG-IFN-α 2a (2.0%) and rIFN-α 2a (2.0%), individually. All interferons have almost the same efficiency and induce about the same activation of the KYN pathway [36]. No patient had a past record of psychiatric treatment, and all were off from depressive symptoms prior to IFN-α treatment. They did not take any antidepressant medications during the study period. At an average of 104.2 ± 15.8 days after the IFN-α administration, some patients presented with apathy, social isolation tendencies, melancholy, depressed mood, and an intention to stop IFN administration. Patients who felt depressed mood were referred for psychiatric

(a) Clinical characteristics of HCV patients

	Depression (−)	Depression (+)
All subjects	30 (male: 20; female:10)	19 (male: 12; female: 7)
Age	54.33 ± 2.06	54.0 ± 2.29
HCV genotype 1b	24 (80%)	15 (78.9%)
HCV genotype 2a	4 (13.3%)	3 (15.8%)
HCV genotype 2b	2 (6.7%)	1 (5.3%)
AST	59.43 ± 5.09	57.47 ± 6.45
ALT	82.68 ± 11.36	69.56 ± 8.65

"Depression (−)": HCV patients without depression, "Depression (+)": HCV patients with depression following IFN-α therapy [47]. HCV, hepatitis C virus; AST, aspartate aminotransferase; ALT, alanine aminotransferase.

(b) The time points of blood sampling

Time points	Depression (−) (mean ± SEM)	Depression (+) (mean ± SEM)	*t*	df	p value
(a) Before the onset of therapy	1–35 d (6.3 ± 1.8 d)	0–22 d (6.7 ± 1.3 d)	0.230	48	0.819
(b) 2 w after the onset of therapy	13–15 d (13.8 ± 0.1 d)	12–15 d (13.6 ± 0.2 d)	0.513	61	0.610
(c) 4 w after the onset of therapy	25–30 d (27.9 ± 0.1 d)	25–29 d (27.6 ± 0.3 d)	0.952	40	0.347
(d) The period of therapy	167–343 d (252.0 ± 15.7 d)	54–337 d (183.4 ± 22.0 d*)	2.592	46	0.013

For all HCV patients, blood was collected before the onset of IFN-α therapy, as well as 2 and 4 weeks after the onset of therapy, and after the end or cessation of therapy. See **Figure 3a** for a detailed blood sampling schedule.*p<0.05 *versus* Depression (−) [47].

Table 1. Clinical information for HCV patients undergoing IFN-α therapy.

evaluation and identified as major depressive disorder (MDD) by a psychiatrist. Nineteen of the HCV patients were diagnosed with depressive symptoms [depression (+)], while 30 of them did not present depressive symptoms [depression (−)]. The diagnosis to verify the incidence of depressive symptoms associated to MDD was made according to the DSM-IV (Diagnostic and Statistical Manual of Mental Disorders fourth edition) and ICD-10 (International Statistical Classification of Disease and Related Health problems-10) base on clinical interviews.

For all HCV patients, blood was collected before the onset of IFN-α therapy as well as 2 and 4 weeks after initiation of treatment. There was a no significant time difference for blood sampling between depression (−) and (+) patients (**Table 1b** and **Figure 3**).

Previous studies suggested that IDO1-mediated TRP metabolism could be implicated in the development of depression, as a side effect of IFN-α therapy in HCV patients. We also found that HCV patients showed decreased TRP and increased KYN concentrations without any changes in KA, AA, and 3-HAA concentrations during IFN-α therapy (**Figure 3b** and **Table 2a**). Furthermore, depression (+) patients presented a higher increase in 3-HK concentration compared to depression (−) patients during treatment (**Table 2a**). Ogawa et al. recently showed that plasma TRP concentration was significantly decreased in MDD patients compared to healthy controls [37]. Teraishi et al. also demonstrated increased KYN metabolites along the TRP-KYN-QUIN pathway, but not the KYN-KA pathway, in MDD patients [38]. Our results showed that the level of 3-HK in the serum significantly increased in depression (+) patients are consistent with these findings. We also investigated the ratios of 3-HK/KA (reflecting neurotoxic indices) [39, 40] and KYN/TRP (reflecting IDO1 activity) in depression (−) and depression (+) HCV patients during IFN-α treatment (**Figure 3c** and **Table 2b**). The ratios of KYN/TRP and 3-HK/KA in both groups increased during treatment. However, in depression (+) patients, the ratios of KYN/TRP and 3-HK/KA increased much larger in depression (−) patients during treatment (**Table 2b**). In these patients, the serum KYN/TRP and 3-HK/KA ratios increased more at the diagnosis of depression, but at 70.3 ± 9.1 days post therapy, they returned to the same levels as before onset of the therapy (data not shown). The severity of depression was not assessed during treatment, using neither the MADRS nor Hamilton Depressing Rating Scale. Therefore, we could not clearly show the direct association between the aggravation of depressive symptoms and changes in TRP metabolites. However, our results suggest that HCV patients with a high sensitivity for IDO1 activation by IFNs are highly susceptible to the depression-related side effects of IFN-α treatment.

4.2. The effects of chronic *Ifn-γ* gene expression on depression-like behavior in mice

We hypothesized that the high induction of IDO1 and the imbalance of TRP metabolites induced by IFNs in humans may be related to psychiatric side effects, such as depression. Previous studies have shown that all three IFNs (IFN-α, -β, and -γ) induce strong IDO1 activity in human peripheral blood mononuclear cells [41, 42]. In contrast, in mouse, IDO1 is induced more markedly by IFN-γ than IFN-α, which has only a weak direct IDO1-stimulatory effect. Therefore, we investigated whether IDO1 activity induced by *Ifn-γ* gene transfer impaired behavior in mice.

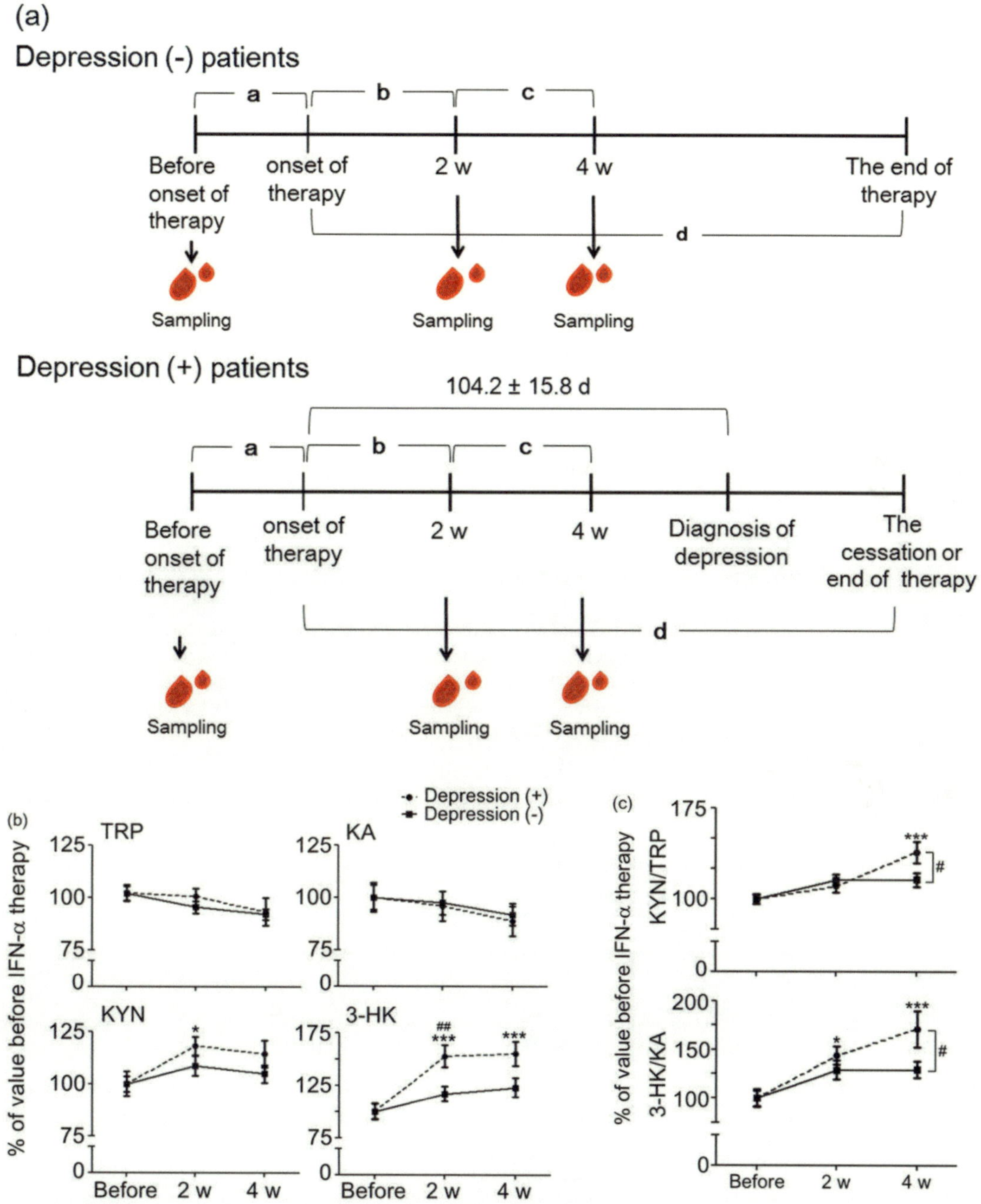

Figure 3. Changes in the levels of serum TRP and its metabolites in HCV patients receiving IFN-α therapy. Original data from Ref. [47]. (a) Schematic depiction of the collection schedule for blood sampling from depression (−) and depression (+) HCV patients. The range of time points and average collection time point (a–d) per group are listed in **Table 1b**. (b) Serum TRP, KYN, KA, and 3-HK concentrations in HCV patients at 2 and 4 weeks after the onset of therapy, expressed as a percentage of the concentration before IFN-α therapy. (c) Serum KYN/TRP and 3-HK/KA ratios in HCV patients are shown as a percentage of values before IFN-α therapy. Rectangles indicate non-depressive HCV patients [Depression (−)] and circles indicate HCV patients with depressive symptoms [Depression (+)]. Each data point represents the mean ± SEM of values obtained from n = 30 depression (−) patients and n = 19 depression (+) patients. $^{*}p<0.05$, $^{***}p<0.001$ *versus* before the onset of IFN-α therapy, $^{\#}p<0.05$, $^{\#\#}p<0.01$ *versus* depression (−) patients. Detailed statistical analyses are shown in **Table 2** [47].

(a) Changes in the levels of serum TRP and its metabolites

	% of value before IFN-α therapy		*t*	df	*p* value
	Depression (–)	**Depression (+)**			
2 w after onset of therapy					
TRP	95.4 ± 2.93	100.5 ± 3.98	0.965	40	0.340
KYN	108.6 ± 4.77	118.1 ± 4.24*	1.200	39	0.237
3-HK	117.0 ± 7.13	152.6 ± 10.4***, $^{\#\#}$	2.886	38	0.006
KA	97.4 ± 5.51	95.9 ± 7.13	0.136	38	0.892
AA	119.9 ± 7.42	115.5 ± 7.11	0.381	41	0.706
3-HAA	102.9 ± 6.53	121.8 ± 12.6	1.452	37	0.155
4 w after onset of therapy					
TRP	92.0 ± 2.55	93.3 ± 6.49	0.213	39	0.833
KYN	104.8 ± 4.38	114.4 ± 6.38	1.204	39	0.236
3-HK	123.0 ± 9.01	155.0 ± 11.5***	2.005	36	0.053
KA	91.9 ± 5.12	88.8 ± 6.98	0.341	40	0.735
AA	107.5 ± 5.32	103.6 ± 11.3	0.361	40	0.720
3-HAA	101.9 ± 6.52	104.5 ± 14.8	0.182	36	0.857

Percent value of serum TRP, KYN, 3-HK, KA, AA, and 3-HAA concentrations in HCV patients at 2 and 4 weeks after the onset of therapy, compared to the concentration (100%) before IFN-α therapy. In the clinical samples, some metabolites were difficult to separate clearly by HPLC. Therefore, the degree of freedom (df) values differ by the measured molecules. "Depression (–)": HCV patients without depression, "Depression (+)": HCV patients with depression.$^{*}p<0.05$,
$^{***}p<0.001$ *versus* before the therapy;
$^{\#\#}p<0.01$ *versus* Depression (–) [47].

(b) Changes in serum KYN/TRP and 3-HK/KA ratios

	% of value before IFN-α therapy		*t*	df	*p* value
	Depression (–)	**Depression (+)**			
2 w after onset of therapy					
KYN/TRP	115.6 ± 4.55	114.1 ± 5.95	0.198	42	0.844
3-HK/KA	129.1 ± 9.52	144.0±9.06*	1.036	39	0.308
4 w after onset of therapy					
KYN/TRP	115.7 ± 5.69	138.3±8.84*,$^{\#}$	2.094	35	0.044
3-HK/KA	129.6 ± 8.67	171.1 ± 18.6***,$^{\#}$	2.325	35	0.026

Serum KYN/TRP reflects IDO1 activity, and 3-HK/KA reflects neurotoxic indices. Both ratios in HCV patients were shown as % of value compared to the value (100%) before IFN-α therapy, at 2 and 4 weeks after the onset of therapy.$^{*}p<0.05$,
$^{***}p<0.001$ *versus* before the therapy;
$^{\#}p<0.01$ *versus* Depression (–) [47].

Table 2. Changes in TRP-KYN pathway in HCV patients undergoing IFN-α therapy.

To conduct this experiment, for murine *Ifn-γ* gene transfer, the plasmid pCpG-Muγ was constructed by inserting a BglII/NheI murine *Ifn-γ* cDNA fragment into the BglII/NheI site of the pCpG-mcs vector (**Figure 4a**). The prepared plasmid pCpG-Muγ was dissolved in normal saline and injected into the tail veins of the mice for over 5 s on day 0. The injection volume was approximately 9% (v/w) of body weight. To eliminate the possibility of tissue damage or inflammation by the hydrodynamic injection, a control plasmid, which was the empty vector without the *Ifn-γ* gene (pCpG-mcs), was injected (0.05 pmol/mouse; IFN-γ transfected (−) mice). A previous study demonstrated that sustained IFN-γ concentrations were observed in mice receiving pCpG-Muγ at a dose of 0.2 pmol/mouse and more than 1000 pg/mL of IFN-γ was detected in the serum from 6 to 31 days after injection of pCpG-Muγ [43]. We also confirmed that the injected plasmid, pCpG-Muγ (IFN-γ transfected (+) mice) significantly increased IDO1 activity in the frontal cortex over a dose of 0.05 pmol/mouse compared to IFN-γ transfected (−) mice (**Figure 4c**). Therefore, the plasmid dose was fixed at 0.05 pmol/mouse for subsequent experiments, which corresponded to 0.10–0.12 μg of DNA/mouse.

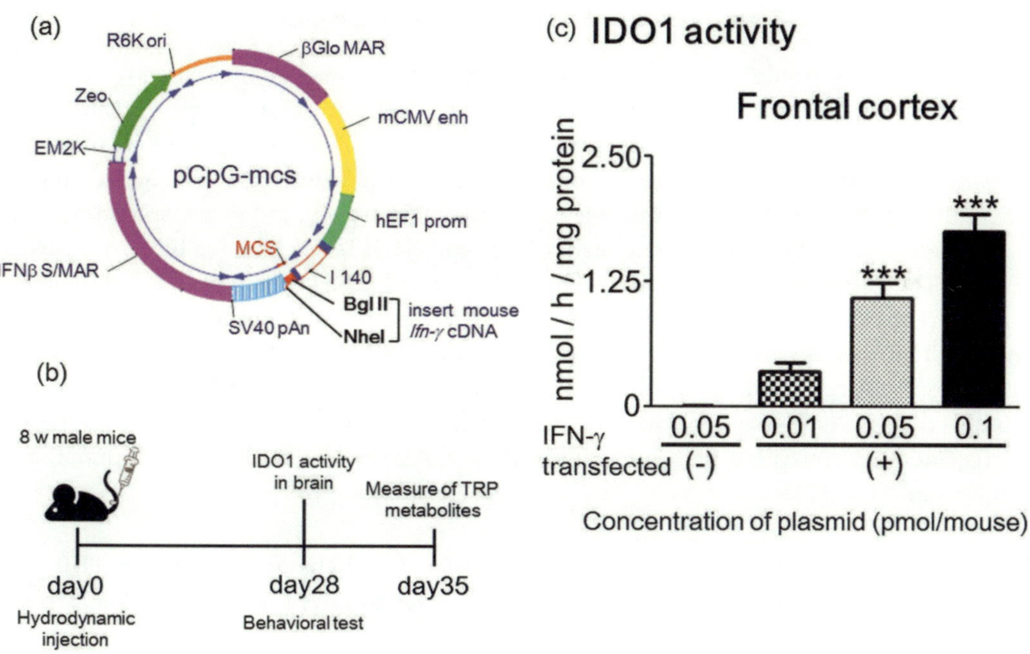

Figure 4. *Ifn-γ* gene transfer. Original data from Ref. [47]. (a) Schematic depiction of the pCpG-Muγ plasmid construct (InvivoGen, San Diego, CA). (b) Schematic depiction of the time schedule for animal experiments. (c) Increase of IDO1 activity in the frontal cortex of mice 28 days after *Ifn-γ* gene transfer [47]. βGlo MAR, β-globin matrix attachment region; mCMV enh, mouse cytomegalovirus enhancer; hEF1 prom, human elongation factor1 promoter; I140, synthetic 5′UTR containing an intron 140; MCS, multi cloning site; SV40 pAn, Simianvirus 40 polyadenylation; IFN-β S/MAR, interferon β gene scaffold/matrix attachment region; EM2K, CpG-free version of the bacterial EM7 promoter; Zeo, Zeocin; R6K ori, R6K origin.

In order to clarify whether the activation of IDO1 by IFN-γ-affected behaviors, three tests, open-field test (OFT), the Y-maze test, and forced swimming test (FST), were performed in mice. Mice were transfected with either a pCpG-mcs plasmid (control vector) that did not contain the *Ifn-γ* gene [IFN-γ-transfected (−) mice] or a pCpG-Muγ plasmid that long-lasting expressed *Ifn-γ* [IFN-γ transfected (+) mice]. No significant differences in locomotor activity of the OFT was observed between IFN-γ transfected (−) and (+) mice. Similarly, in the Y-maze test, no significant differences in the alternation behavior were detected between the two groups of mice. However, in the FST, immobility time was significantly longer in IFN-γ-transfected (+) mice (**Figure 5a**). Our findings strongly suggest that IDO1 induction by IFN-γ is a critical factor in depression-like behaviors but not in short-term memory or locomotor activity in mice.

4.3. Changes in the levels of TRP and its metabolites in the serum and frontal cortex of mice following chronic Ifn-γ gene expression

In order to further elucidate the relationship between the IDO1-induced KYN pathway and the development of depression-like behavior in mice transfected with the pCpG-Muγ plasmid, we measured TRP metabolites in the serum and frontal cortex of these mice.

The serum and the frontal cortex were corrected from mice immediately following behavioral testing to determine the levels of TRP, KYN, KA, 3-HK, 3-HAA, and AA (**Figure 5b** and **c**). The concentration of serum TRP was significantly decreased in IFN-γ transfected (+) mice compared to IFN-γ-transfected (−) mice. In contrast, the levels of serum KYN and 3-HK were significantly increased in the IFN-γ-transfected (+) mice (**Figure 5b**). In the frontal cortex, IFN-γ transfected (+) mice had significantly higher KYN and 3-HK levels than the IFN-γ-transfected (−) mice. The TRP and KA levels in the frontal cortex tended to be lower in the IFN-γ-transfected (+) mice (**Figure 5c**). The activation of IDO1 by *Ifn-γ* gene transfer significantly modified the levels of TRP and its metabolites not only in the serum, but also in the frontal cortex of mice. These results suggest that an alternative explanation for the participation of IDO1 in IFN-γ-induced depression-like behavior is the generation of neuroactive TRP metabolites. This interpretation is consistent with our clinical data and previous studies by O'Connor et al. and Wichers et al. [32, 35].

4.4. The effects of Ido1 gene-deficiency on depression-like behavior, changes in TRP metabolism, 5-HT, and its turnover in the frontal cortex of mice following chronic Ifn-γ gene expression

Additionally, we evaluated the role of IDO1 in the development of depression-like behavior after *Ifn-γ* gene transfer using *Ido1* gene knockout (KO) mice, and determined the levels of TRP metabolites in the frontal cortex.

The increase in time spent in an immobile posture in the *Ifn-γ*-transfected (+)/wild type mice was significantly improved in *Ido1* KO mice (**Figure 6a**). In wild type mice, *Ifn-γ* gene transfer significantly increased the concentrations of KYN and 3-HK in the frontal cortex by 4.7- and 2.5-fold, respectively. In contrast, *Ido1* KO mice withdrew these changes in *Ifn-γ* gene transfer

http://dx.doi.org/10.5772/intechopen.71013

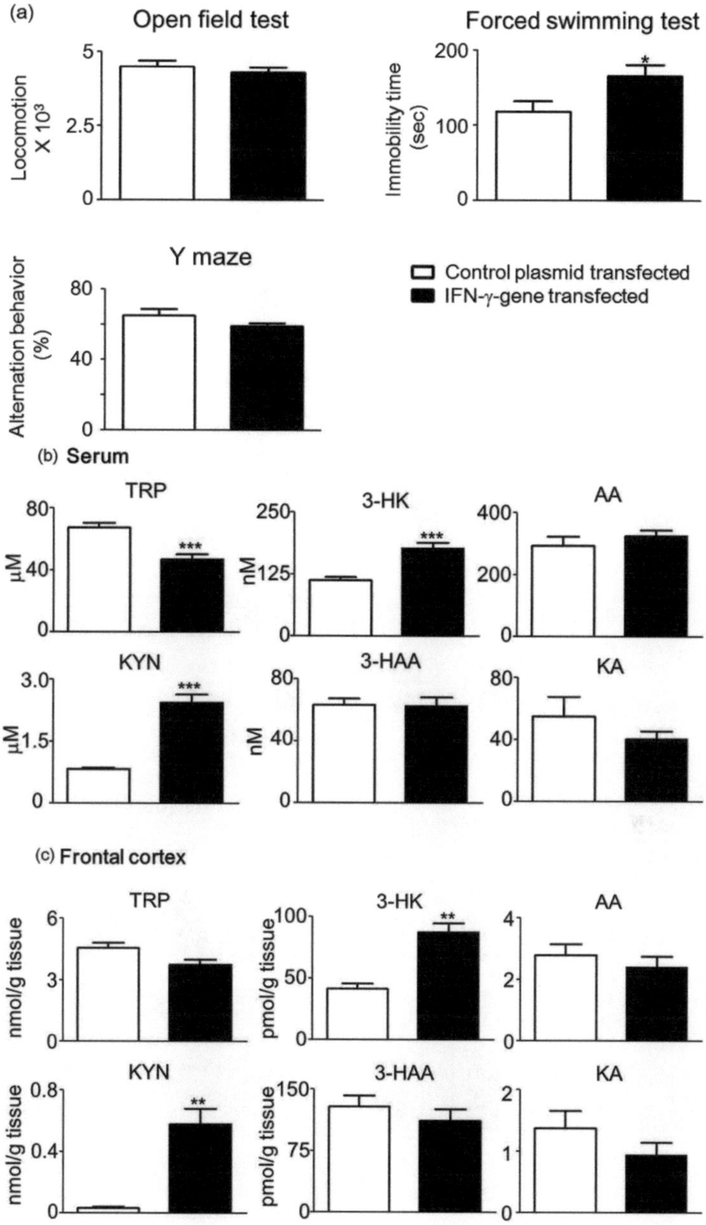

Figure 5. The effect of chronic *Ifn-γ* gene expression on the TRP-KYN pathway and depression-like behavior in mice. Original data from Ref. [47]. (a) Behavioral changes in mice 28 days after *Ifn-γ* gene transfer. Open field test shows locomotor activity of mice in a novel environment. Y-maze test shows short-term memory. Forced swim test shows depression-like behavior. Immobility time was significantly increased in IFN-γ-transfected (+) mice, compared to IFN-γ-transfected (−) mice. The open bar shows IFN-γ-transfected (−) mice, and the closed bar shows IFN-γ-transfected (+) mice. Each column represents the mean ± SEM (n = 9–16). *p <0.05 *versus* IFN-γ-transfected (−) mice. (b) (c) Changes in the levels of TRP and its metabolites in the serum and frontal cortex of mice after *Ifn-γ* gene transfer. TRP-KYN metabolite concentrations were determined in the serum (b) and the frontal cortex (c) of mice 35 days after *Ifn-γ*-gene transfer. The open bar shows IFN-γ-transfected (−) mice, and the closed bar shows IFN-γ-transfected (+) mice. Each column represents the mean ± SEM (n = 15–20). **p<0.01, ***p<0.001 *versus* IFN-γ-transfected (−) mice [47].

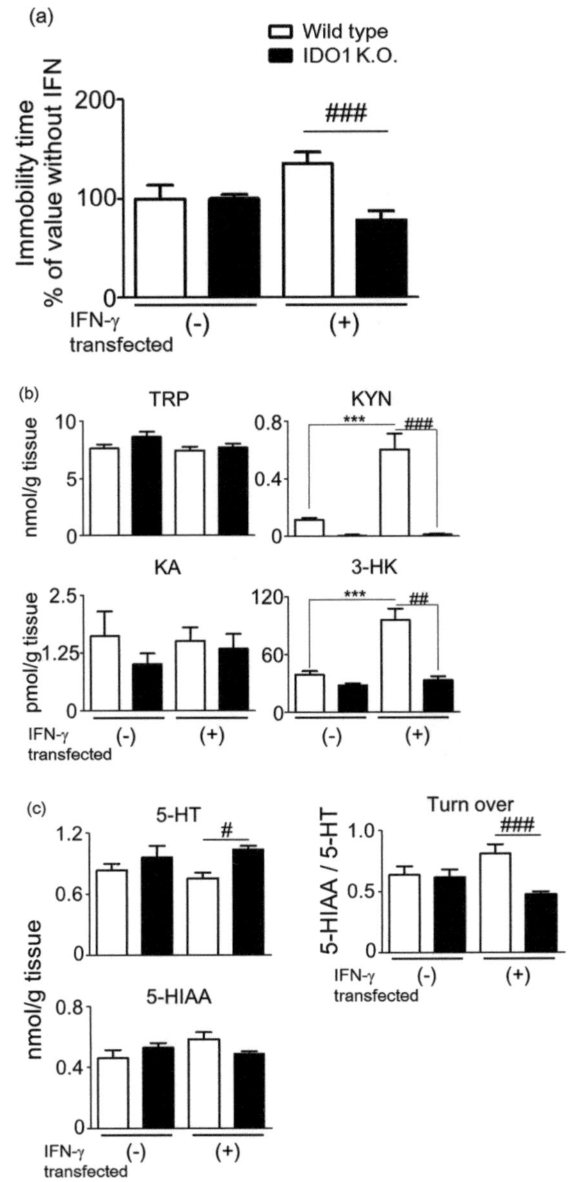

Figure 6. The effects of *Ido1* gene-deficiency on depression-like behavior, changes in TRP metabolism, 5-HT, and its turnover in the frontal cortex of mice following chronic *Ifn-γ* gene expression. Original data from Ref. [47]. (a) Abnormal behavior in a forced swimming test after *Ifn-γ* gene transfer in mice was improved in *Ido1* gene deficient mice. The Y axis shows the percent value of immobility time in IFN-γ-transfected (+) mice, compared to the time (100%) in IFN-γ-transfected (−) mice (n = 8–15). (b) The level of TRP metabolites in the frontal cortex of mice 35 days after *Ifn-γ*-gene transfer (n = 6–15). (c) The amount of 5-HT, 5-HIAA, and 5-HIAA/5-HT ratio as an index of serotonin turnover in the frontal cortex of mice 35 days after *Ifn-γ*-gene transfer (n = 6–15). The open bar represents wild type and the closed bar, *Ido1* gene deficient mice. IFN-γ-transfected (−) mice were injected with the control plasmid (pCpG-mcs), and IFN-γ-transfected (+) mice were injected with the IFN-γ-expressing pCpG-Muγ plasmid. Each column represents the mean ± SEM. *$p<0.05$, ***$p<0.001$ *versus* IFN-γ-transfected (−) wild type mice, #$p<0.05$, ##$p<0.01$, ###$p<0.001$ *versus* IFN-γ-transfected (+) wild type mice [47].

mice (**Figure 6b**). The levels of KYN and 3-HK in the frontal cortex after *Ifn-γ* gene transfer were considerably lower in *Ido1* KO mice than in wild type mice. Even though we cannot exclude the possibility that genetic deficient in *Ido1* and the resulting modifications in TRP metabolites could influence other behavioral tests, our results clearly demonstrate that *Ido1* KO mice do not show depression-like behavior and do not intensify TRP metabolites after *Ifn-γ* gene transfer.

Other studies have emphasized that the 5-HT pathway is also relevant to depression. In a clinical study, it has been shown that levels of TRP and 5-hydroxytryptophan, a precursor of 5-HT, were significantly decreased from their baseline levels in the serum of HCV patients during IFN-α therapy [44]. Thus, we speculate that biological mechanisms underlying the IFN-α treatment induced-depressive symptoms are linked not only to the activated IDO1 and KYN pathway but also to a dysfunction of the 5-HT system. To clarify on the basis of the neurotransmitter changes in depression-like behavior after *Ifn-γ* gene transfer, we measured the concentrations of 5-HT and its metabolite 5-hydroxyindoleacetic acid (5-HIAA) in the frontal cortex of wild type and *Ido1* KO mice (**Figure 6c**). We showed that *Ifn-γ* gene transfer produced a trend toward increased 5-HIAA levels in wild type mice but not in *Ido1* KO mice. These results indicated that *Ifn-γ* gene transfer induced a potential increase in IDO1-induced 5-HT turnover. A raised 5-HT turnover suggests a process by which the availability of 5-HT to be released by neurons is decreased to compensate for neuronal dysfunction associated with depression-like behavior promoted by *Ifn-γ* gene transfer. Correspondingly, previous clinical studies have shown that brain 5-HT turnover is significantly increased in MDD patients without medication and decreased following selective serotonin reuptake inhibitors (SSRI) therapy [45, 46].

Taken together, an alternative interpretation for the involvement of IDO1 in IFN-γ-induced depression-like behavior may be that depression is related to not only the generation of neuroactive TRP metabolites but also to the alteration of serotoninergic neurotransmission.

5. Conclusion

The levels of TRP metabolites in the serum of HCV patients changed significantly. In particular, the increase in serum 3-HK concentration in depressive HCV patients was much larger than that in HCV patients without depressive symptoms. The ratios of serum KYN/TRP, reflecting IDO1 activity, and 3-HK/KA were increased in depressive and non-depressed HCV patients with therapy. However, the increase in serum KYN/TRP and 3-HK/KA ratios in depressive patients was much higher than that of non-depressive HCV patients. When the *Ifn-γ* gene was transfected into normal mice, depression-like behavior significantly increased. Additionally, *Ifn-γ* gene transfer to mice induced dramatic changes in TRP metabolite concentrations in the serum and the prefrontal cortex. On the other hand, genetic deletion of *Ido1* abrogated the enhanced depression-like behavior after *Ifn-γ* gene transfer. In conclusion, our results clearly show that IDO1 is a critical molecular regulator of the depressive pathology induced as a side effect of interferon therapy. Moreover, the depressive symptoms are induced via increases in degradation of TRP and neuroactive metabolites along the KYN pathway, which finally changes in the alternation of 5-HT turnover. Our findings suggest that inflammatory pathways that lead to the activation of IDO1 may be a novel therapeutic target in patients suffering from inflammation-associated depression, for example, HCV or cancer therapy. Our results also suggest the monitoring of TRP-KYN metabolites during immunotherapy might assist in predicting the onset risk of depression as a side effect in these patients. However, further insight into the role of each downstream KYN pathway metabolite in the pathological process is needed to understand, and to clarify the relationship with complex neurotransmitters.

Acknowledgements

This work was supported by Grant-in Aid for Scientific Research of YM (26860368 and 16K08948).

Author details

Yuki Murakami[1*] and Yukio Imamura[1,2]

*Address all correspondence to: ymurakam@mail.doshisha.ac.jp

1 Organization for Research Initiatives and Development, Doshisha University, Kyoto, Japan

2 Department of Traumatology and Acute Critical Medicine, Osaka University Graduate School of Medicine, Osaka, Japan

References

[1] Asnis GM, De La Garza R 2nd. Interferon-induced depression in chronic hepatitis C: A review of its prevalence, risk factors, biology, and treatment approaches. Journal of Clinical Gastroenterology. 2006;**40**(4):322-335. DOI: 10.1097/01.mcg.0000210099.36500.fe

[2] Hoofnagle JH. Hepatitis C: The clinical spectrum of disease. Hepatology. 1997;**26**(3 Suppl 1):15S-20S. DOI: 10.1002/hep.510260703

[3] Pockros PJ. Developments in the treatment of chronic hepatitis C. Expert Opinion on Investigational Drugs. 2002;**11**(4):515-528. DOI: 10.1517/13543784.11.4.515

[4] Strader DB, Wright T, Thomas DL, Seeff LB, American Association for the Study of Liver Diseases. Diagnosis, management, and treatment of hepatitis C. Hepatology. 2004;**39**(4):1147-1171. DOI: 10.1002/hep.20119

[5] Dorr RT. Interferon-alpha in malignant and viral diseases: A review. Drugs. 1993;**45**(2): 177-211

[6] Miyaoka H, Otsubo T, Kamijima K, Ishii M, Onuki M, Mitamura K. Depression from interferon therapy in patients with hepatitis C. The American Journal of Psychiatry. 1999;**156**(7): 1120. DOI: 10.1176/ajp.156.7.1120

[7] Musselman DL, Lawson DH, Gumnick JF, Manatunga AK, Penna S, Goodkin RS, et al. Paroxetine for the prevention of depression induced by high-doseinterferon alfa. The New England Journal of Medicine. 2001;**344**(13):961-966. DOI: 10.1056/NEJM200103293441303

[8] Bonaccorso S, Marino V, Puzella A, Pasquini M, Biondi M, Artini M, et al. Increased depressive ratings in patients with hepatitis C receiving interferon-alpha-based immunotherapy are related to interferon-alpha-induced changes in the serotonergic system. Journal of Clinical Psychopharmacology. 2002;**22**(1):86-90

[9] Fischer CW, Eskelund A, Budac DP, Tillmann S, Liebenberg N, Elfving B, et al. Interferon-alpha treatment induces depression-like behaviour accompanied by elevated hippocampal quinolinic acid levels in rats. Behavioural Brain Research. 2015;**293**:166-172. DOI: 10.1016/j.bbr.2015.07.015

[10] Raison CL, Dantzer R, Kelley KW, Lawson MA, Woolwine BJ, Vogt G, et al. CSF concentrations of brain tryptophan and kynurenines during immune stimulation with IFN-alpha: relationship to CNS immune responses and depression. Molecular Psychiatry. 2010;**15**(4):393-403. DOI: 10.1038/mp.2009.116

[11] Steiner J, Walter M, Gos T, Guillemin GJ, Bernstein HG, Sarnyai Z, et al. Severe depression is associated with increased microglial quinolinic acid in subregions of the anterior cingulate gyrus: evidence for an immune-modulated glutamatergic neurotransmission? Journal of Neuroinflammation. 2011;**8**:94. DOI: 10.1186/1742-2094-8-94

[12] Chung RT, Gale M Jr, Polyak SJ, Lemon SM, Liang TJ, Hoofnagle JH. Mechanisms of action of interferon and ribavirin in chronic hepatitis C: Summary of a workshop. Hepatology. 2008;**47**(1):306-320. DOI: 10.1002/hep.22070

[13] Takaoka A, Yanai H. Interferon signalling network in innate defence. Cellular Microbiology. 2006;**8**(6):907-922. DOI: 10.1111/j.1462-5822.2006.00716.x

[14] Gale M Jr, Foy EM. Evasion of intracellular host defence by hepatitis C virus. Nature 2005;**436**(7053):939-945, DOI: 10.1038/nature04078.

[15] Sen GC. Viruses and interferons. Annual Review of Microbiology. 2001;**55**:255-281. DOI: 10.1146/annurev.micro.55.1.255

[16] Cook DN, Pisetsky DS, Schwartz DA. Toll-like receptors in the pathogenesis of human disease. Nature Immunology. 2004;**5**(10):975-979. DOI: 10.1038/ni1116

[17] Iwasaki A, Medzhitov R. Toll-like receptor control of the adaptive immune responses. Nature Immunology. 2004;**5**(10):987-995. DOI: 10.1038/ni1112

[18] McCormick CJ, Challinor L, Macdonald A, Rowlands DJ, Harris M. Introduction of replication-competent hepatitis C virus transcripts using a tetracycline-regulable baculovirus delivery system. The Journal of General Virology. 2004;**85**(Pt 2):429-439. DOI: 10.1099/vir.0.19676-0

[19] Sumpter R Jr, Loo YM, Foy E, Li K, Yoneyama M, Fujita T, et al. Regulating intracellular antiviral defense and permissiveness to hepatitis C virus RNA replication through a cellular RNA helicase, RIG-I. Journal of Virology 2005;**79**(5):2689-2699, DOI: 10.1128/JVI.79.5.2689-2699.2005

[20] Li K, Chen Z, Kato N, Gale M Jr, Lemon SM. Distinct poly(I-C) and virus-activated signaling pathways leading to interferon-beta production in hepatocytes. The Journal of Biological Chemistry. 2005;**280**(17):16739-16747. DOI: 10.1074/jbc.M414139200

[21] Yoneyama M, Kikuchi M, Natsukawa T, Shinobu N, Imaizumi T, Miyagishi M, et al. The RNA helicase RIG-I has an essential function in double-stranded RNA-induced innate antiviral responses. Nature Immunology. 2004;**5**(7):730-737. DOI: 10.1038/ni1087

[22] Fitzgerald KA, McWhirter SM, Faia KL, Rowe DC, Latz E, Golenbock DT, et al. IKKepsilon and TBK1 are essential components of the IRF3 signaling pathway. Nature Immunology. 2003;**4**(5):491-496. DOI: 10.1038/ni921

[23] Kanazawa N, Kurosaki M, Sakamoto N, Enomoto N, Itsui Y, Yamashiro T, et al. Regulation of hepatitis C virus replication by interferon regulatory factor 1. Journal of Virology. 2004;**78**(18):9713-9720. DOI: 10.1128/JVI.78.18.9713-9720.2004

[24] Murray PJ. The JAK-STAT signaling pathway: input and output integration. Journal of Immunology. 2007;**178**(5):2623-2629

[25] Honda K, Takaoka A, Taniguchi T. Type I interferon [corrected] gene induction by the interferon regulatory factor family of transcription factors. Immunity. 2006;**25**(3):349-360. DOI: 10.1016/j.immuni.2006.08.009

[26] Menkes DB, MacDonald JA. Interferons, serotonin and neurotoxicity. Psychological Medicine. 2000;**30**(2):259-268

[27] Capuron L, Ravaud A, Neveu PJ, Miller AH, Maes M, Dantzer R. Association between decreased serum tryptophan concentrations and depressive symptoms in cancer patients undergoing cytokine therapy. Molecular Psychiatry. 2002;**7**(5):468-473. DOI: 10.1038/sj.mp.4000995

[28] Hassanain HH, Chon SY, Gupta SL. Differential regulation of human indoleamine 2,3-dioxygenase gene expression by interferons-gamma and -alpha. Analysis of the regulatory region of the gene and identification of an interferon-gamma-inducible DNA-binding factor. The Journal of Biological Chemistry. 1993;**268**(7):5077-5084

[29] Lawson MA, Parrott JM, McCusker RH, Dantzer R, Kelley KW, O'Connor JC. Intracerebroventricular administration of lipopolysaccharide induces indoleamine-2,3-dioxygenase-dependent depression-like behaviors. Journal of Neuroinflammation. 2013;**10**:87. DOI: 10.1186/1742-2094-10-87

[30] O'Connor JC, Andre C, Wang Y, Lawson MA, Szegedi SS, Lestage J, et al. Interferon-gamma and tumor necrosis factor-alpha mediate the upregulation of indoleamine 2,3-dioxygenase and the induction of depressive-like behavior in mice in response to

bacillus Calmette-Guerin. The Journal of Neuroscience. 2009;**29**(13):4200-4209. DOI: 10.1523/JNEUROSCI.5032-08.2009

[31] O'Connor JC, Lawson MA, Andre C, Briley EM, Szegedi SS, Lestage J, et al. Induction of IDO by bacille Calmette-Guerin is responsible for development of murine depressive-like behavior. Journal of Immunology. 2009;**182**(5):3202-3212. DOI: 10.4049/jimmunol.0802722

[32] O'Connor JC, Lawson MA, Andre C, Moreau M, Lestage J, Castanon N, et al. Lipopolysaccharide-induced depressive-like behavior is mediated by indoleamine 2,3-dioxygenase activation in mice. Molecular Psychiatry. 2009;**14**(5):511-522. DOI: 10.1038/sj.mp.4002148

[33] Salazar A, Gonzalez-Rivera BL, Redus L, Parrott JM, O'Connor JC. Indoleamine 2,3-dioxygenase mediates anhedonia and anxiety-like behaviors caused by peripheral lipopolysaccharide immune challenge. Hormones and Behavior. 2012;**62**(3):202-209. DOI: 10.1016/j.yhbeh.2012.03.010

[34] Vecsei L, Beal MF. Influence of kynurenine treatment on open-field activity, elevated plus-maze, avoidance behaviors and seizures in rats. Pharmacology, Biochemistry, and Behavior. 1990;**37**(1):71-76

[35] Wichers MC, Koek GH, Robaeys G, Verkerk R, Scharpe S, Maes M. IDO and interferon-alpha-induced depressive symptoms: a shift in hypothesis from tryptophan depletion to neurotoxicity. Molecular Psychiatry. 2005;**10**(6):538-544. DOI: 10.1038/sj.mp.4001600

[36] Malaguarnera M, Laurino A, Di Fazio I, Pistone G, Castorina M, Guccione N, et al. Neuropsychiatric effects and type of IFN-alpha in chronic hepatitis C. Journal of Interferon & Cytokine Research. 2001;**21**(5):273-278. DOI: 10.1089/107999001300177457

[37] Ogawa S, Fujii T, Koga N, Hori H, Teraishi T, Hattori K, et al. Plasma L-tryptophan concentration in major depressive disorder: new data and meta-analysis. The Journal of Clinical Psychiatry. 2014;**75**(9):e906-e915. DOI: 10.4088/JCP.13r08908

[38] Teraishi T, Hori H, Sasayama D, Matsuo J, Ogawa S, Ishida I, et al. Personality in remitted major depressive disorder with single and recurrent episodes assessed with the Temperament and Character Inventory. Psychiatry and Clinical Neurosciences. 2015;**69**(1):3-11. DOI: 10.1111/pcn.12218

[39] Johansson AS, Owe-Larsson B, Asp L, Kocki T, Adler M, Hetta J, et al. Activation of kynurenine pathway in ex vivo fibroblasts from patients with bipolar disorder or schizophrenia: cytokine challenge increases production of 3-hydroxykynurenine. Journal of Psychiatric Research. 2013;**47**(11):1815-1823. DOI: 10.1016/j.jpsychires.2013.08.008

[40] Savitz J, Drevets WC, Smith CM, Victor TA, Wurfel BE, Bellgowan PS, et al. Putative neuroprotective and neurotoxic kynurenine pathway metabolites are associated with hippocampal and amygdalar volumes in subjects with major depressive disorder. Neuropsychopharmacology. 2015;**40**(2):463-471. DOI: 10.1038/npp.2014.194

[41] Carlin JM, Borden EC, Sondel PM, Byrne GI. Biologic-response-modifier-induced indoleamine 2,3-dioxygenase activity in human peripheral blood mononuclear cell cultures. Journal of Immunology. 1987;**139**(7):2414-2418

[42] Werner-Felmayer G, Werner ER, Fuchs D, Hausen A, Reibnegger G, Wachter H. Induction of indoleamine 2,3-dioxygenase in human cells in vitro. Advances in Experimental Medicine and Biology. 1991;**294**:505-509

[43] Mitsui M, Nishikawa M, Zang L, Ando M, Hattori K, Takahashi Y, et al. Effect of the content of unmethylated CpG dinucleotides in plasmid DNA on the sustainability of transgene expression. The Journal of Gene Medicine. 2009;**11**(5):435-443. DOI: 10.1002/jgm.1317

[44] Comai S, Cavalletto L, Chemello L, Bernardinello E, Ragazzi E, Costa CV, et al. Effects of PEG-interferon alpha plus ribavirin on tryptophan metabolism in patients with chronic hepatitis C. Pharmacological Research. 2011;**63**(1):85-92. DOI: 10.1016/j.phrs.2010.10.009

[45] Barton DA, Esler MD, Dawood T, Lambert EA, Haikerwal D, Brenchley C, et al. Elevated brain serotonin turnover in patients with depression: Effect of genotype and therapy. Archives of General Psychiatry. 2008;**65**(1):38-46. DOI: 10.1001/archgenpsychiatry.2007.11

[46] Sullivan GM, Oquendo MA, Huang YY, Mann JJ. Elevated cerebrospinal fluid 5-hydroxyindoleacetic acid levels in women with comorbid depression and panic disorder. The International Journal of Neuropsychopharmacology. 2006;**9**(5):547-556. DOI: 10.1017/S1461145705006231

[47] Murakami Y, Ishibashi T, Tomita E, Imamura Y, Tashiro T, Watcharanurak K, et al. Depressive symptoms as a side effect of Interferon-alpha therapy induced by induction of indoleamine 2,3-dioxygenase 1. Scientific Reports. 2016;**6**:29920. DOI: 10.1038/srep29920

Chapter 4

Application of Pharmacokinetics in Early Drug Development

Katherine Dunnington, Natacha Benrimoh, Christine Brandquist, Nadia Cardillo-Marricco, Mike Di Spirito and Julie Grenier

Additional information is available at the end of the chapter

http://dx.doi.org/10.5772/intechopen.74189

Abstract

The intention of this chapter is to provide an overview of how pharmacokinetics, also termed PK, is applied in early drug development. While there are many readily available printed and web accessible sources on pharmacokinetics, its technical terms, model definitions, and calculation methods; how the science of pharmacokinetics is used in specific situations, namely early drug development are not as readily covered. In fact, the reader will see that the continual theme in this chapter is that a small amount of pharmacokinetic data and its interpretation in the first nonclinical or clinical study is important in obtaining additional pharmacokinetic, safety, and efficacy information for the next study. The role of PK in the three phases of clinical drug development is described as well as the types of early Phase 1 studies where PK determinations are important. The PK measurements in the first in humans study (FIH) provide a tentative confirmation of safety at the measured exposures from the tested dose levels. Even if exposures from a given dose change due to food-effects, drug–drug interaction, drug-disease interactions, or use in a special population, safety can be assessed by bridging these results to the initial safety or efficacy exposures.

Keywords: pharmacokinetics, drug development, compartmental modeling, non-compartmental pharmacokinetics, non-clinical pharmacokinetics

1. Introduction

The intention of this chapter is to provide an overview of how pharmacokinetics, also termed PK, is applied in early drug development. Since, PK is defined as the study of the effects of a living organism on an administered drug, the majority of pharmacokinetic studies involve the measurement of a specific compound in an easily sampled physiological fluid, like blood, plasma, serum and on occasion, in saliva. Excreted substances are also measured in urine or feces. In some rarer situations, measurements are made with more invasive sampling methods, such as a tissue biopsy, cerebral spinal fluid, bronchoalveolar lavage fluid, or middle ear effusion fluid. Regardless of the sample type, the measured concentrations are regarded as indicative of the concentrations at the specific site of action for the drug. Even excreted drug data can be used to describe the PK within the body; drug excretion rates into urine are recognized as proportional to plasma concentrations at midpoints of the collection interval, and amounts of drug in urine and feces can give some idea of excretion pathways. Series of drug concentrations measured in biological fluids over an adequate amount of time give the pharmacokinetic scientist a 'window' into the body, and by analyzing the time course of concentrations, information on the unseen drug in the various body compartments can be inferred. Thus, applied pharmacokinetics are useful in various types of pharmacological evaluations, be it for academic purposes, clinical research (inside and outside of drug development), or in clinical medicine (individualized dosing and therapeutic drug monitoring) [1–3].

While there are readily available printed and online materials on pharmacokinetic topics such as its technical terms, model definitions and calculation methods [4–5]; there are some gaps when it comes to how the science of pharmacokinetics is used in drug development. Several authors however, have touched on various aspects and a reader of this chapter may gain additional knowledge by consulting them [6–8]. Most healthcare workers and scientists are relatively familiar with the clinical pharmacology and medicine package inserts which include a pharmacokinetic section of an approved drug's labeling. This section of the package insert gives the general information that has been gleaned from large amounts of research and helps the practitioner or scientist understand the general absorption, distribution, metabolism, and elimination of a given therapeutic agent. In essence, this is only a short summary of what is known about this drug. Not readily apparent from the short summary is the role that pharmacokinetics had from the start of a drug's development through its approval journey. Through the application of pharmacokinetics, the maximum information can be extracted from data when only a few subjects are available as in a first in human (FIH) clinical study and then this information is applied to the design and interpretation of the next study during the drug's development phase. Furthermore, even before the first clinical human study is conducted, pharmacokinetic and toxicological data from animals can be used to predict human pharmacokinetics and to assist in the determination of a safe starting dose and the optimal study design. In fact, the reader will note that the continual theme in this chapter is that pharmacokinetic data and their interpretation in the first study is important in obtaining additional pharmacokinetic, safety, and efficacy information a subsequent study, and so on, throughout the drug development process. In the following pages, various types of PK evaluations and/or studies are described.

2. Pharmacokinetics and early drug development

Clinical drug development, meaning drug research in human subjects, is generally described in three phases, each comprised of a number of different clinical studies, Phases 1, 2, and 3, (see

http://dx.doi.org/10.5772/intechopen.74189

Figure 1) [9, 10]. However these three phases do not encompass the entirety of the research for any given new drug: nonclinical research starts prior to Phase 1, and post-marketing studies (sometimes referred to as Phase 4) continue after Phase 3 and medicines regulatory agency's approval. Once a new chemical entity (NCE), a new molecular entity (NME), a new biological entity (NBE), a new active substance (NAS) or a new therapeutic entity (NTE) [11], also called investigational product (IP), or in general for this chapter, a new drug, is identified and the minimum *in vitro* and animal data are gathered, and after filing an application with the appropriate regulatory agency, a promising substance can start clinical research [12]. For sake of clarity, an overview of the three phases of studies is given below and the roles of PK data are highlighted.

Phase 1 studies (some exploratory studies are also called Phase 0) in clinical drug development are described as the initial introduction of the drug into humans, in small numbers of healthy subjects (if appropriate), starting at lower doses and escalating as safe to therapeutic ranges and super therapeutic ranges if possible. The reasons for studying higher doses, if deemed safe to do so, can be multi-faceted. Confirming safety at higher doses helps determine a margin of safety around the efficacious doses, and aids in determining the clinical relevance of any drug–drug- and drug-disease-interactions, or special population differences that may be elucidated later. Pharmacokinetics over a wider range leads to the ability to correlate drug effects (therapeutic or adverse) with drug exposure, and to characterize these relationships [13]. The aforementioned safety margin also allows the drug sponsor some flexibility in determination of the final marketed dose if necessary. Phase 1 also includes specific studies designed to study special populations, such as the elderly, children, in people

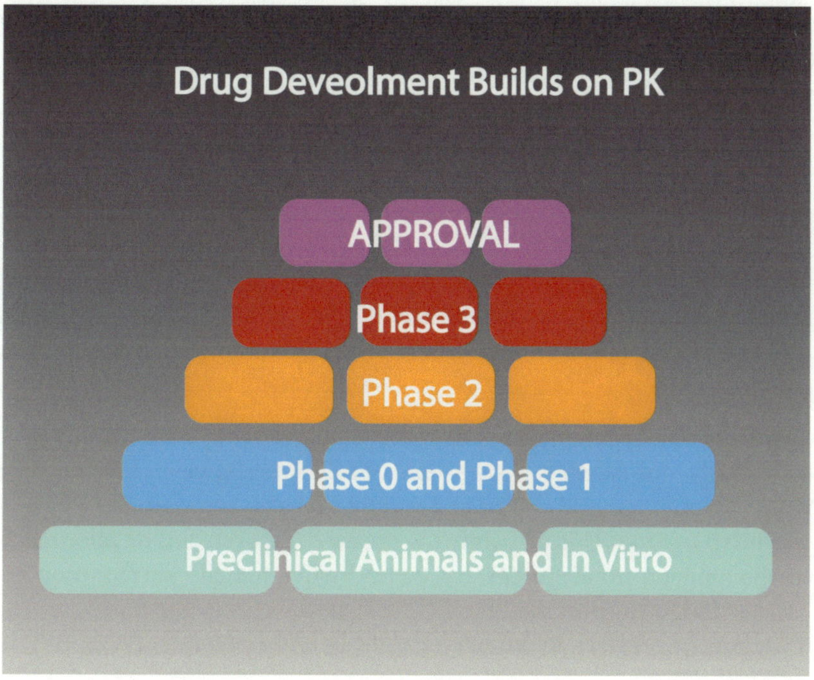

Figure 1. Phases of drug development built on pharmacokinetics.

with hepatic or renal impairment. In these studies, pharmacokinetic endpoints are the primary goal, allowing relatively small studies (low numbers of subjects) to inform the future Phase 2 and 3 studies and marketing after approval. The results of these studies are reflected in the approved drug's labeling, where warnings about the use in certain disease-states or dosage adjustments are communicated.

In Phase 2 studies of clinical drug development, the objective is not only to determine that a drug continues to be safe but that it remains to be safe when used in patients with the disease it is intended for to treat. The information gathered in Phase 2 serves the dual purpose of studying safety and efficacy while providing proof to the sponsor that the drug is worthy of further development. The pivotal Phase 2 study for continuation of Phase 2 and/or starting Phase 3 is often called 'Proof of Concept (POC).' The value of PK measurements in Phase 2 adds another layer of understanding how the body processes the drug; these studies determine differences in PK data between categories of patients, namely those with the targeted disease and normal healthy volunteers. Sometimes patients will have higher or lower exposures of a drug due to the difference in ability to absorb a drug, or the drug may be eliminated differently due to the disease state. In general, the more the patient is affected/weakened by the disease, the more PK will differ from healthy subjects. Knowledge of the PK in the patient population forms a bridge to knowledge of safety and perhaps efficacy gathered in Phase 1. Phase 2 PK facilitates any need for dose adjustments to achieve safety or efficacy. PK correlations with efficacy can begin in earnest once patient data is available; this data along with the Phase 1 data is modeled and simulations using those models assist in choosing the Phase 3 dose ranges.

Phase 3 in clinical drug development consists of several large studies in patient populations designed to collect further safety data, to observe possible adverse events which occur only rarely, to continue to evaluate efficacy and compare with current therapies for the indication, and to guide its use once approved and on the market. However, clinical research does not necessarily come to a halt at the end of Phase 3. After approval and marketing, additional studies may be run by the sponsor to establish marketing claims and to seek new indications. Adverse event data are continually collected to identify even rarer adverse events not uncovered in Phase 3. Phase 3 PK data is usually performed only as a few samples in many subjects or complete profiles in a subset of subjects; this data is for confirmatory purposes, used in correlation with efficacy or adverse events. This data is added to the ongoing modeling (discussed later in Section 3.1) to discern sources of variability in the PK data from the patient population.

The above descriptions of each phase of drug development may seem as though each phase precedes sequentially, one starting after the end of the other; however this may not always be the case. While typically the end of Phase 2 commences the beginning of Phase 3, the other phases may overlap in time. This is mainly to conserve research and development resources. For instance, the longer animal studies and reproductive toxicity studies may not run until the results are needed to support the Phase I and II studies for drugs that may require longer treatment durations or research in women of child-bearing potential (WOCBP), respectively

[14]. A thorough Phase I study to determine QTc prolongation and potential for cardiac arrhythmias (if not characterized already in earlier studies) should not be run until some idea of the clinical doses and exposures are determined and after a few studies have shown some promise for the drug's future approval.

3. Pharmacokinetic analyses

Pharmacokinetic analyses types can be broken into two general approaches: compartmental and non-compartmental. Non-compartmental analyses are a series of calculations that estimate the exposures and elimination properties of a drug with very few assumptions about the particular mechanisms involved. Non-compartmental exposure parameters (such as area under the concentration-time curve (AUC) and the maximum exposure (Cmax) can be calculated and are interpretable when no other PK information is available; these parameters indicate the amount of drug in the body and for how long it is there, and the peak concentration that is achieved.

Compartmental methods can be described as the determination of a mathematical expression, or model, which adequately describes the PK of a given drug. On the most basic level, these models consist of the mathematical description representing the body as one or a series of hypothetical volume compartments which drug distributes into and out of, or from which it is eliminated. These models not only describe the PK properties of a drug, but can be predictive of PK at different dose levels or administration conditions. Complex models aid in the elucidation of smaller processes which make up the PK in its entirety, such as the rate and capacity of the different metabolism pathways involved in a drug's elimination.

3.1. Compartmental pharmacokinetics

The process of fitting PK data to a given mathematical description, or model, is known as compartmental modeling. This modeling is carried out with specialized software applications and [15, 16] **Figure 2** shows the simplest one-compartment PK model where drug is introduced by an intravenous bolus injection into a representative volume compartment and the differential and integrated equations that can be fitted to actual data to determine the values of the constants as defined. Multiple-compartment PK models, such as a 2-compartment model, or a 3-compartmental model, commonly describe a concentration-time course adequately, but more complex models may contain more compartments. The mathematical models are based on the processes which move drug into or out of the compartments; these may be a constant rate of infusion or elimination (a zero-order kinetic process) or concentration-driven diffusion processes (first-order kinetics) or by saturable active transport or metabolic processes (Michaelis–Menten kinetics), or combinations thereof [17–19]. The intention of a compartmental model can be as straightforward as to find the simplest model which describes the PK and predicts drug exposures under new conditions, like a higher dose, or when administered in multiple doses over time, or when administered under a different route

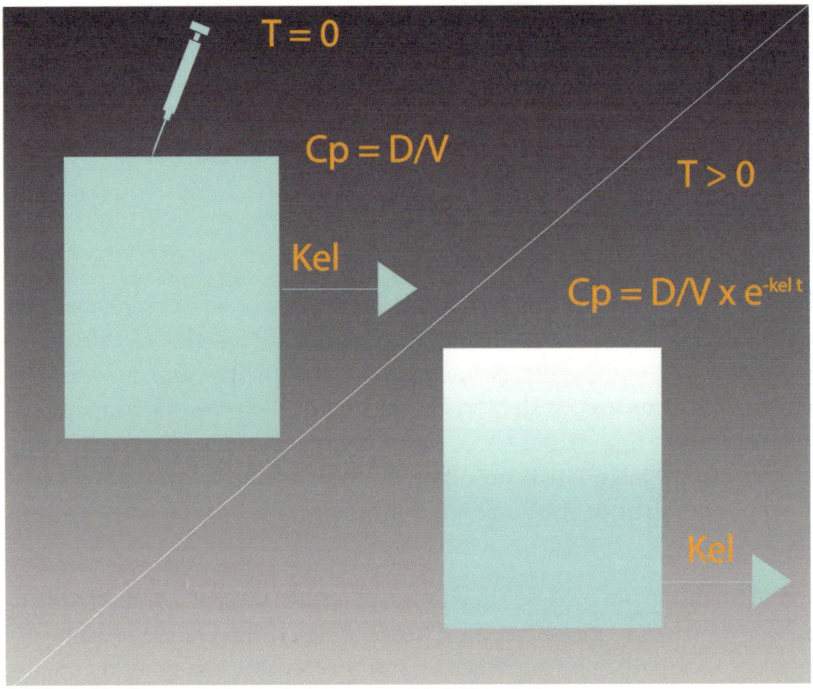

Figure 2. One-compartment pharmacokinetic model. graphic presentation of a one-compartment PK model with an intravenous bolus injection of dose (D) into a single central compartment of volume V, with a first-order elimination rate of kel. Where Cp is the concentration in the compartment which decreases over time (t). The model is described by a single differential (1) $dCp/dt = D/V \times (-kel)$. The integrated Eq. (2) is $Cp = (D/V)\ e^{-kelT}$. Secondary parameter CL (clearance) is calculated by Eq. (3) $CL = V^*kel$.

of administration. However, sometimes the purpose may be more complex, to elucidate additional processes such as metabolism mechanisms or drug effects, and these models may contain many compartments.

Compartmental modeling in the very early stages of drug development might be used for supplemental information or to set the initial assumptions for further additional modeling later in the drug development program; known as population pharmacokinetics [20]. Population pharmacokinetics (termed in the industry as 'Pop PK') is the systemic analysis of compiled data from specific studies or from the entire drug development program. These analyses are used to better understand the concentration-time course of the drug and to explain potential sources of PK variability. These models take either sparse PK data (limited numbers of samples) from large numbers of subjects and patients, or both, and/or rich sampling data (full serial PK sampling profiles) from early PK studies, and often incorporate development of individual patient covariates (e.g., BMI, race, genotypes, concomitant medications, disease status, etc.) to predict exposure and effects in individual patients. **Figure 3** shows that this type of analysis not only allows individual patient predictions, but also provides average PK parameters for the population. A population PK approach is also useful in clinical research situations where

http://dx.doi.org/10.5772/intechopen.74189

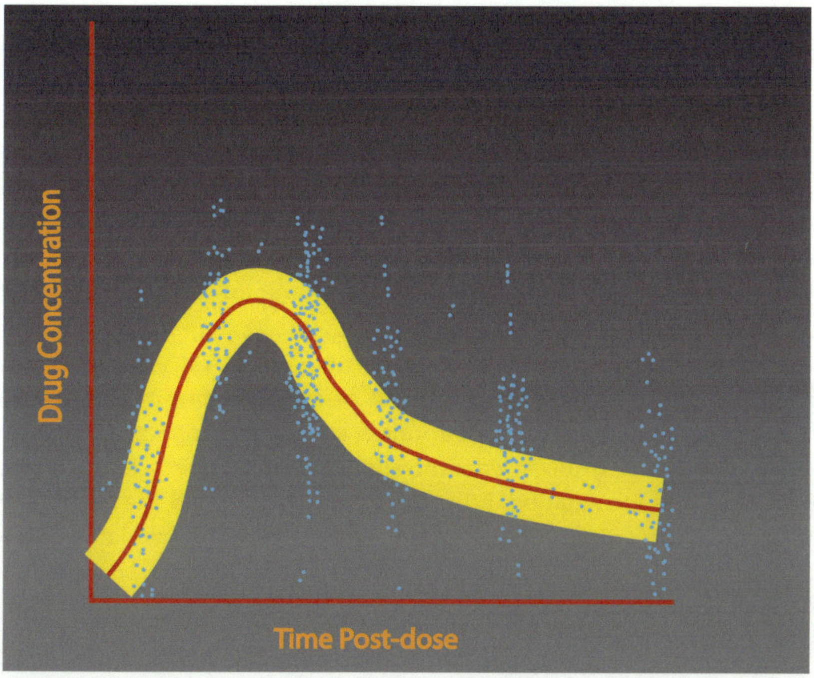

Figure 3. Population pharmacokinetics. Population model predictions (solid line) with 95% CI (shaded area) with observed data (circles).

ethics, patient safety, and/or patient comfort limit the number of PK samples that can be collected, such as in neonates, pediatrics, and patients with advanced diseased states.

Compartmental and non-compartmental (to be discussed Section 3.2) PK parameter estimates tend to vary within (intra-patient variability) and between individuals (inter-patient variability), with some drugs having more variability than others. Commonly these estimates vary by at least ±15–20% in normal volunteers which can make interpretations challenging, especially when only a few subjects have been evaluated. PK estimates in patient populations typically have even more variability. Population pharmacokinetics, once data is obtained in enough patients and subjects, can help identify and characterize the various sources of variability.

3.2. Non-compartmental pharmacokinetics

Non-compartmental pharmacokinetics include a number of calculations performed with a series of PK samples usually with plasma- or serum-concentration-time data. These parameters provide a model-free description of how the drug is dispersed and eliminated from the body. These types of analysis can be done very quickly with limited numbers of subjects, where in compartmental or population modeling can take quite some time to build a model. Since no assumptions of which type of compartmental model fits the data best are required, a non-compartmental approach is applied in most Phase I PK studies, and is quite useful in understanding the drug and indexing its exposure, determining the clinical dose, and designing the final marketed dosage form. The PK parameters obtained from non-compartmental analyses are illustrated in **Figure 4**. Cmax, the peak concentration gives researchers a maximum drug exposure and is also dependent on the absorption rate for extravascular administrations, while the time of Cmax, Tmax, is also indicative of the rate of absorption, but one must understand drug elimination is also occurring at this time. The log-linear slope at the end of the concentration-time curve can be used to estimate the terminal elimination rate constant and the terminal elimination half-life, assuming the curve is well characterized and the PK exhibits first-order elimination. Too short of a sampling interval or limitations of the bioanalytical method may result in missing the terminal elimination phase, so in some cases this slope may be more representative of drug distribution. By calculating an area under the concentration-time curve, called AUC, an index of overall exposure is obtained, and this exposure is independent of the shape of the curve, be it the sharp increase of an intravenous injection with a high Cmax, or lower concentrations observed over a longer amount of time after a slow-release oral formulation. From AUC calculations and the terminal elimination rate constant, estimations volume of distribution and clearance, abbreviated as V and CL, for intravenous doses, or after extravascular doses abbreviated V/F and CL/F, unadjusted for the bioavailable, F, can be made.

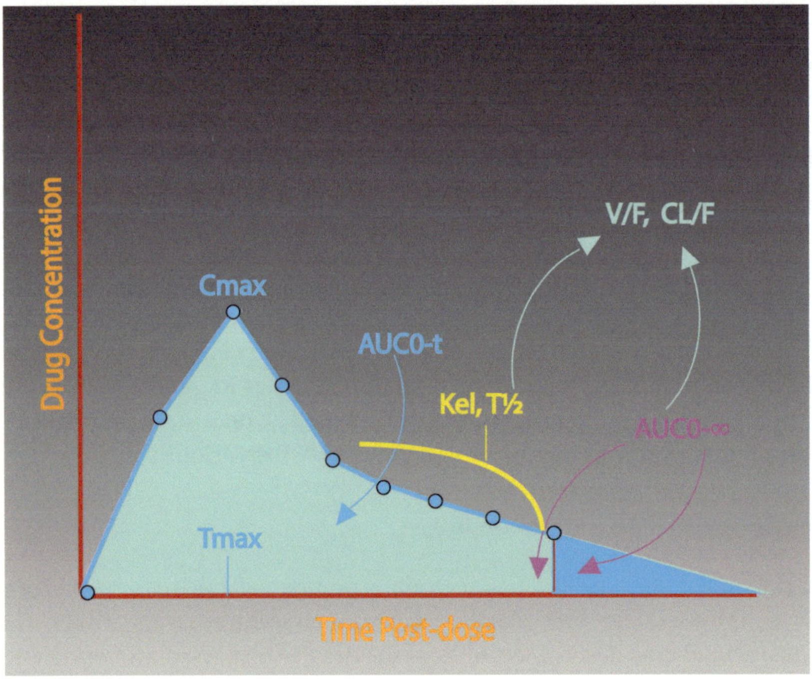

Figure 4. Non-compartmental model parameters. Cmax = peak concentration, Tmax = time of peak concentration, kel = negative terminal slope from ln concentration versus time regression, T1/2 = 0.693/kel (apparent terminal elimination half-life) AUC0-t = Area un the concentration-time curve from 0 to the last quantifiable concentration estimated by the trapezoidal rule, AUC0-∞ = Area under the curve extrapolated to infinity (AUC0-t + Cp(t)/kel, CL/F = Dose/AUC0-∞ (after a single dose), V/F = apparent volume of distribution after an extravascular dose, calculated by CL/F / kel.

4. Nonclinical pharmacokinetics

Before an investigational drug is ever administered to a human subject, an immense amount of animal and in vitro data are gathered. For example, tests in cell lines and/or animal models are used to determine the potential of the drug's therapeutic action. Other in vitro tests can screen for safety, such as in hERG (Human ether-a-go-go Related Gene) expressed cells, to determine a drug's potential to interact with the potassium channel, I_{KR}, and cause cardiac arrhythmias [21]. Ultimately, single- and repeat-dose toxicity studies, also called 'toxicokinetic or TK' studies, in rodents and at least 1 non-rodent species are needed to support the investigation of the drug in humans [14]. While these studies are mandated by regulatory agencies, they are also useful in the design of the FIH study for a drug's development program. Depending on the type of drug and its apparent risk, several methods of determining the starting dose based on observed toxicity at dose levels can be used. These methods range from simple adjustment and allometric scaling of the non- observed adverse effect level (NOAEL) in the most sensitive animal species studied, with a safety margin [22]. to complex scaling modeling to predict human exposures from animal data. For particularly risky compounds, the starting dose is sometimes carefully based on the minimum biologically active concentration and its associated dose level, also called the minimum effective dose (MED) [23].

Sometimes detailed PK in animals is available, but generally the PK data from animal studies come from the toxicoketinetic studies. In these studies, the goal is to determine exposure for correlation with toxicity, but qualitative expectations of how the drug will behave in a human are conceived. It would be expected, but not guaranteed, that a quickly absorbed and quickly eliminated drug would also act similarly in humans. Useful predictions of a drug's human PK can be made using computer modeling techniques, called PBPK (physiological based pharmacokinetic modeling) interspecies scaling, which take different species' capacities of absorption, body distribution, and metabolic/excretion into account and simulate PK concentrations based on an analogous human model [21, 24–26].

Nonclinical studies are also important for providing an idea of the mechanism of the drug's metabolism, whether any cytochrome P 450 enzymes are involved, and identification of metabolites which could be important in humans [27]. Metabolites identified in animals that represent 10% of drug circulating material need to be monitored in toxicology studies and later in clinical studies if still a significant metabolite, is disproportionately produced in humans, or if it is biologically active [28]. In vitro experiments with hepatic enzyme preparations and various chemical probes identify which CYP 450 enzymes are potentially active in the metabolism of a drug. Once these are determined, potential drug-drug interaction pathways are realized; this information is then used to design Phase I drug-drug interaction studies to characterize the clinical significance of these possible interactions in. In vitro experiments also provide the identities of drug-transporters which may move drug into or out of various organs in the body. Drug–drug interactions can also be mediated by inhibition or competition within these transporter systems [29].

5. Early clinical studies with primary endpoints of safety

Earlier this chapter described the primary objective of Phase I as determining safety in a small number of subjects before the introduction of the drug into patients. This remains true, but for the purposes of this chapter, Phase I studies will be described as studies whereby safety measurements are the primary endpoint (or finding) and where primary endpoints are PK-related.

5.1. First in human studies

The main purpose of the first in human clinical study (FIH) for a drug is to test that it is safe, meaning that subjects are monitored for signs of toxicity, especially those indicating risk of mortality or morbidity. Tolerability, the ability of a patient to use the drug for its intended indication, without unacceptable, non-life-threatening adverse events that would require discontinuation of treatment, is also an important consideration. Risk-to-benefit ratios are considered when determining the required tolerability and risks of toxicity; a drug for a life-saving, unmet clinical need, such as cancer, would be considered for approval even if it carries more risk than a drug for a self-limiting or non-life-threatening disease, such as the common cold. From the animal data discussed above, researchers have a good idea of the types of toxicity and at what exposures they may occur for a given drug, yet the first human study is critical in confirming the drug's potential for toxicity in a human. PK in a FIH is therefore very informative, telling us not just if toxicity occurs, but at what exposure that toxicity correlates with.

5.2. Single-ascending-dose studies (SAD)

Typically, the FIH study is the single-ascending dose study, where small numbers of subjects are dosed carefully with either the drug or placebo, and safety is monitored by recording adverse events, clinical laboratory measurements, vital signs, electrocardiograms, and additional tests depending on concerns raised in the animal studies or from the known pharmacology. Once a small dose is administered and considered to be safe, then a higher dose (typically 2–3 times higher than the starting dose) is administered to a new group of subjects which is then considered before a higher yet dose is given. The escalation schedule for ascending doses needs to be considered carefully, using smaller increments of increase with higher risk drugs, the predicted therapeutic range for the drug, and the levels of exposure where toxicity was seen in animals [30]. Study protocols for drugs considered to be high risk or of narrow therapeutic range may have stopping criteria based on PK as well as safety. Some study protocols will set an upper limit on PK parameters of exposure that are not to be exceeded in the study. The escalation schedule or planned doses may be revised depending upon the outcome of the previously dosed groups. Unexpected toxicity may require lowering the dose and subsequent doses; lower than expected exposure (if assessed before the study finishes) might require increasing the planned doses or accelerating the dose escalation.

The design of the FIH study will incorporate animal data or interspecies scaling predictions to determine when and how long blood (usually plasma or serum) should be sampled for PK measurements. Ideally, to characterize a PK profile, sampling would be optimized to capture absorption rates, peak concentrations, distribution and elimination phases, and would minimally be 2–3 times the elimination half-life, preferably 4–5 times the elimination half-life. Sometimes at lower dose levels this is difficult due to the limitation of the bioanalytical method used to measure drug concentrations.

When PK information is needed for dose escalation a common practice is to perform interim PK analyses as the study progresses, where the PK is examined in one group before proceeding to the next higher dose level group. This is a time sensitive process where careful planning with logistics between the clinic conducting the study, sample shipment, the laboratory analyzing the samples, the scientist performing the PK calculations, and sometimes a data safety monitoring board (DSMB) who will review the data and make a determination along with the sponsor and principal investigator in charge of clinic conduct. Once at least two dose levels have been administered, the scientist will use the data obtained to date in order to determine if the increase in exposure is proportional to the increase in dose (dose proportionality) and if so to predict what exposures might be at the next dose level, given that dose proportionality continues to the next dose. If dose proportionality is not seen (the PK may be described as 'nonlinear') [31], and the increase is higher than proportional to the increase in dose, escalation to higher dose levels should proceed with caution, as saturation of a metabolic or elimination pathway could lead to sharp increases in PK concentrations with only a small increase in dose. If PK concentrations are less than proportional to the increase in dose, indicating a saturation in the absorption process, then the dose escalation schedule may need to be revisited in order to achieve target exposures.

5.3. Multiple-ascending-dose studies (MAD)

PK information gained in the single-ascending dose assessment of a drug development program is used further in the design of the next clinical study, which for most drugs is the multiple-ascending dose study. Because most drugs need to be given repeatedly over time, safety information for continuous use is needed. In this study, the drug is administered for the number of doses required (based on the single-dose PK) to reach steady-state levels, the highest exposure a given drug regimen will achieve, where the given drug exhibits first-order elimination (**Figure 5**). Again, the main purpose of the study is to determine safety at maximum exposures, but PK at these exposures is applicable to the design of the next study in the drug development program. Steady-state levels depend upon the half-life, the dose, and how often the drug is given (also called the frequency of administration). If PK properties after a single dose are known, then the number of repeated doses given at equal intervals for a duration of approximately 5 times the half-life will reach predictable steady-state levels. Confirmation of steady-state in this type of study is usually assessed by determining if trough (predose) concentrations for the last few doses are approaching a constant value; [32] this also helps confirm that the half-life observed after single doses was based upon the elimination phase, that the PK is indeed first order, and is or is not 'linear' over time. Linear or nonlinear, the single- and multiple-dose studies in Phase I not only determine safety at a certain exposure, but the relationship of dose to exposure, leading to predictability to adequately achieve target exposures further along in Phases II and III.

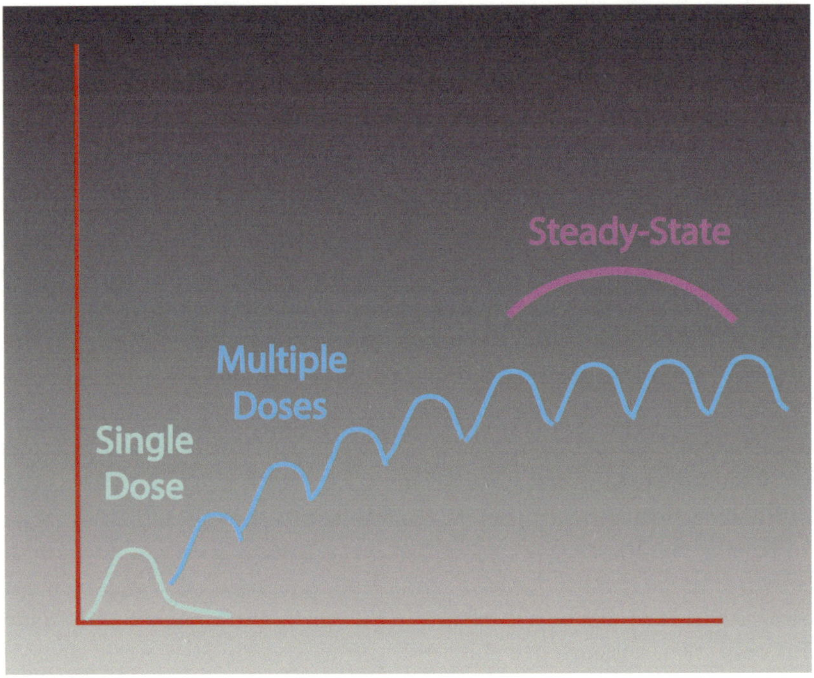

Figure 5. Single dose and steady-state pharmacokinetics.

It should be noted that the single- and multiple-dose studies are not always run in two separate studies. Depending upon the sponsor, type of drug, its PK qualities, and how much dose-limiting toxicity is expected, these assessments may all be performed under a single study protocol [33]. These studies are termed SAD/MAD studies, and may be designed in two parts, a single-dose and a multiple-dose part to follow when the first is completed or partially completed. Sometimes the study is designed for the sequential groups to get a single dose followed by a washout period where they are monitored, and then the same group will be started on multiple doses at the same level as the first dose for a period of time expected to reach steady state. Safety and or PK is examined for that group, and if deemed safe, then the dose is escalated in the next group.

6. Early clinical studies with primary PK endpoints

Once the SAD and MAD studies have confirmed acceptable safety to proceed further into Phase 1, several types of studies are conducted where PK endpoints are the primary objective, and continued collection of safety data is only secondary. These studies determine the effects of other drugs, diseases, and patient qualities on the PK of the drug in relatively small numbers of subjects, reducing the risk to patients in the Phase 2 and 3 studies, and ultimately informing the marketed use of the drug.

6.1. Food effect studies

One of the most important PK studies for an orally administered (and sometimes with inhaled drugs where some drug is swallowed) is the food-effect study. An experienced clinical pharmacokineticist will say that the absence of a food effect on the rate or extent of a drug's absorption is rare, and looking at many drugs, most have some difference in absorption between fed and fasted states. Food-effect information is typically not clear from nonclinical studies in most programs, as animals are usually fed ad libitum or on a regular schedule in toxicology studies. A food effect can be somewhat predicted for a specific drug, with knowledge of its solubility, its lipophilicity, and pH dependence on ionization and partitioning, but a human study is required to confirm the extent of the food-effect [34]. Since food in the stomach can affect gastric pH and potentially bind to a drug, and food and/or its fat content can affect gastric emptying time, the probability of some effect on absorption is high. A food effects range from very subtle changes in just Tmax or Cmax, to several-fold increases or decreases in overall exposure, to ultimately where a lipophilic drug might be totally unabsorbed without a minimum of dietary fat. PK parameters, especially Cmax, Tmax, and AUC, can characterize this difference with only a single dose of drug, in a crossover study design, where each subject is administered the drug with and without food. Many drug development programs strive to get this information as early as possible to determine the optimal dosing conditions, and is often part of the SAD, MAD, or SAD/MAD study protocol.

The purpose of the food-effect PK study is to determine if a difference occurs, and if this difference is clinically significant. If found to be clinically significant, that is that food decreases absorption enough to make it less effective, or that it increases absorption enough to cause toxicity. If the PK shows a clinically significant food effect, adjustment of the therapeutic dose and/or instructions on how the drug should be administered will be included in the approved drug labeling. The type of drug is also important in this decision, as commonly food may delay Tmax and decrease Cmax, but if only the extent of exposure (AUC) is important for the drug's efficacy, then the food effect might not be clinically relevant.

6.2. PK studies in special populations

Once the pharmacokinetic behavior of a drug and its initial safety is confirmed in normal healthy volunteers in the early Phase 1 studies, additional Phase 1 studies are performed to determine if PK differs in various special populations [35]. A simple special population study can be used to bridge the entire drug development program of a drug for one population to apply to another population. An example would be a drug developed in Japanese populations that is then intended to also be marketed in the US. Most small molecule drugs are investigated in subjects with hepatic or renal impairment [36, 37], and depending on the drug's intended use, additional studies in elderly, obese, certain racial/ethnic groups, or others are performed. While safety is monitored in these studies, the PK endpoints allow inference of safety and efficacy that has been determined in previous studies. In other words, if age does not appear to affect the PK of a drug, it is well accepted that the previous safety findings will also likely apply, in general, if the drug is used without regard to age. In hepatic and renal impairment, plasma proteins, such as albumin, can be lower than in healthy subjects, so free drug concentrations are often examined to determine if any PK differences are related to the differences in binding, or if increased free drug concentrations might result in any drug effect differences [38]. These studies are often single-dose PK studies in the special group and in healthy volunteers of similar demographics. PK parameters of exposure are key in the between-group comparisons; however, elimination rates and absorption rates are also important.

6.3. Drug-Drug interaction studies

As mentioned previously, nonclinical studies are key in screening a drug for potential drug–drug interactions (DDIs). Once the cytochrome P450 enzymes and transporters for which a new drug is a substrate, an inhibitor, or can induce expression, are identified, clinical studies are performed to confirm, quantitate, and determine clinical significance of any DDI. It would be tedious and cost prohibitive to test every possible DDI, so appropriate probes [39] (other drugs which are known CYP or transporter substrates, inhibitors, or inducers) are chosen to be co-administered and PK measured to determine if a clinically relevant DDI through a specific metabolism or transporter pathway exists [40]. Without PK measurements in this type study, it would take large numbers of subjects to study a drug–drug interaction with safety endpoints only, however with PK, a small number of subjects' exposures to one or both drugs can determine if there is a safety risk by examining previous PK measurements and correlated safety findings. These study designs may differ depending upon the potential interaction, but usually the drug under development is dosed to steady-state at a therapeutic dose. Often these studies are conducted with 12–24 healthy subjects confined to a research clinic, and consist of a fixed treatment sequence for all subjects. An example of a common design would be where the probe drug is administered alone, followed by a washout period, then the multiple doses of the investigational drug are given until steady-state levels are reached, then the probe drug is co-administered. PK of the probe drug is measured to determine if the PK is affected. The sequence could be reversed if the investigational drug is hypothesized to be affected by the probe drug. Two-way DDI designs are also used to determine the two drugs affect each other. The primary PK endpoints are generally Cmax and AUCs to determine if peak or overall exposure differ due to a DDI, but Tmax and elimination rates are helpful in determining if the mechanism is due to decreased metabolism or a change in absorption.

Interpretation of the PK data for these studies is often straightforward; if a DDI increases exposure of a drug, depending upon its safety profile, to a degree that toxicity could develop, or decreases exposure enough that efficacy would be lost, then warnings will be issued in the approved labeling. Occasionally unexpected results in these studies are seen such that relating the results to specific enzymes or transporters becomes difficult, especially when multiple enzymes or unknown transporters are involved. In such instances, the characterization of DDIs helps in the design of Phase 2 and 3 studies where a study protocol excludes patients taking certain medications, and allow the safe investigation in patient populations.

6.4. Radiolabeled drug studies

A concern for a small molecule drug in development is the question of whether the drug is readily removed from the body completely, and how that complete elimination occurs. Less so is whether the drug might accumulate in specific tissues in an undesired way. Along with the question of how a drug is eliminated, another question is what metabolites are formed and how are they excreted. These questions are answered with PK studies using radiolabeled drug, which is commonly called the 'ADME' or 'Mass Balance' study [41]. These studies usually include only 6–8 healthy males given a single dose and confined to a research clinic until most of the drug-related radioactivity has been recovered in urine and/or feces. An easily measurable dose of the study drug is administered along with a small amount of the drug that is radiolabeled, usually with carbon 14 (^{14}C), and sometimes with tritium (^{3}H). PK of unlabeled drug and radioactivity in blood and plasma are measured, and total radioactivity are measured in complete urine and feces collections. These studies can be quite long, as the measurements continue and subjects are confined until only small amounts of radioactivity are excreted in urine/feces each day. The advantage of measuring radioactivity is that it represents the total amounts of drug-related material in blood/plasma, urine, and feces. The drawback for total radioactivity measurements is that it is non-specific. However, comparing unlabeled unchanged drug levels and total radioactivity levels allows the scientist to gauge the amount of metabolites that are circulating and their collective PK behavior. A second aspect of these studies are the determination of the identity of the metabolites and their quantities in plasma, urine and feces by radio chromatography, also known as metabolic profiling. Since the drug was radiolabeled, different chemical entities resulting from the breakdown of the drug in the body can be identified as they will also be radiolabeled. The amounts of radioactivity recovered in urine and feces are totaled, and summed, for the determination of mass balance, i.e. the amount of radioactivity administered is expected to be nearly equal to the radioactivity excreted.

The distribution of the drug and its metabolites (as measured by radioactivity) into erythrocytes is another important aspect of the ADME study, and goes along with the question of drug accumulating in tissues. By measuring radioactivity concentrations in whole blood and in plasma, it is possible to determine if the drug-related material binds to or collects in erythrocytes [42].

7. Summary

The above overview has shown that pharmacokinetics is an integral part of drug development, and a critical part of early drug development. At the beginning of Phase 1 in the development program only animal data is available; hence, what is known through pharmacokinetic measurements in those animal studies is applied in designing Phase 1 human studies. This chapter outlined the importance of pharmacokinetic data in drug development overall and in specific types of early clinical studies. The PK measurements in the FIH study provide confirmation of safety at the measured exposures from the tested dose levels. Even if exposures from a given dose change due to food-effects, drug–drug interaction, drug-disease interactions, or use in a special population, safety can be associated and risks assessed by bridging these results to the initial safety or efficacy exposures. Throughout the drug development program, pharmacokinetics is a tool used to link exposure to efficacy and safety, and it assists in the determination of dosages of marketed drugs; for this reason, PK data are an important part of the information provided to clinicians.

Author details

Katherine Dunnington*, Natacha Benrimoh, Christine Brandquist, Nadia Cardillo-Marricco, Mike Di Spirito and Julie Grenier

*Address all correspondence to: katherine.dunnington@celerionlcom

Celerion, Lincoln, Nebraska, USA

References

[1] Jacob S, Nair AB. An updated overview on therapeutic drug monitoring of recent antiepileptic drugs. Drugs in R&D. 2016;**16**(4):303-316

[2] Freeman K, Saunders MP, Uthman OA, Taylor-Phillips S, Connock M, Court R, et al. Is monitoring of plasma 5-fluorouracil levels in metastatic / advanced colorectal cancer clinically effective? A systematic review. BMC Cancer. 2016;**16**:523

[3] Burton ME. Applied Pharmacokinetics & Pharmacodynamics : Principles of Therapeutic Drug Monitoring. 4th ed. Vol. xvii. Philadelphia: Lippincott Williams & Wilkins; 2006. p. 867

[4] Gibaldi M. Biopharmaceutics and Clinical Pharmacokinetics. 4th ed. Vol. x. Philadelphia: Lea & Febiger; 1991. p. 406

[5] Bourne DWA. Pharmacokinetics and Biopharmaceutics Advanced Course Internet2017 [updated 2017 October 30; cited 2017 October 30]. Available from: https://www.boomer.org/c/p4/

[6] Nishant T, Sathish KD, Arun K, Phaneendra M. Role of pharmacokinetic studies in drug discovery. Journal of Bioequivalence and Bioavailability. 2011;**3**(11):263-267

[7] Chien JY, Friedrich S, Heathman MA, de Alwis DP, Sinha V. Pharmacokinetics/pharmacodynamics and the stages of drug development: Role of modeling and simulation. The AAPS Journal 2005;**7**(3):E544-E559

[8] Walker DK. The use of pharmacokinetic and pharmacodynamic data in the assessment of drug safety in early drug development. British Journal of Clinical Pharmacology. 2004;**58**(6):601-608

[9] Dimasi JA. Risks in new drug development: Approval success rates for investigational drugs. Clinical Pharmacology and Therapeutics. 2001;**69**(5):297-307

[10] Nwangwu PU. Concepts and Strategies in New Drug Development. Vol. xiv. New York: Praeger; 1983. p. 265

[11] Branch SK, Agranat I. "New drug" designations for new therapeutic entities: New active substance, new chemical entity, new biological entity, new molecular entity. Journal of Medicinal Chemistry. 2014;**57**(21):8729-8765

[12] How Drugs are Developed and Approved. Internet: Food and Drug Administration; 2017 [updated 2015 August 18; cited 2017 December 10]. Available from: https://www.fda.gov/Drugs/DevelopmentApprovalProcess/HowDrugsareDevelopedandApproved/default.htm

[13] Garnett C, Bonate PL, Dang Q, Ferber G, Huang D, Liu J, et al. Scientific white paper on concentration-QTc modeling. Journal of Pharmacokinetics and Pharmacodynamics. 2017

[14] Guidance for Industry, M3(R2) Nonclinical Safety Studies for the Conduct of Human Clinical Trials and Marketing Authorization for Pharmaceuticals. January 2010 ed: Division of Drug Information, Center for Drug Evaluation and Research; 2010

[15] Bourne DWA. Pharmacokinetic Software https://www.pharmpk.com/soft.html Bourne DWA; 2017

[16] Shargel L, Yu ABC. Applied Biopharmaceutics & Pharmacokinetics. 7th ed. New York: McGraw-Hill Education; 2016

[17] Mumenthaler MS, Taylor JL, Yesavage JA. Ethanol pharmacokinetics in white women: Nonlinear model fitting versus zero-order elimination analyses. Alcoholism, Clinical and Experimental Research. 2000;**24**(9):1353-1362

[18] Buclin T, Nicod M, Kellenberger S. Elimination Kinetics https://sepia.unil.ch/pharmacology/index.php?id=94: CENTEF of the University of Lausanne; 2017 [updated July 2009]

[19] Benet LZ. General treatment of linear mammillary models with elimination from any compartment as used in pharmacokinetics. Journal of Pharmaceutical Sciences. 1972;**61**(4):536-541

[20] Ette EI, Williams PJ. Population pharmacokinetics I: Background, concepts, and models. The Annals of Pharmacotherapy. 2004;**38**(10):1702-1706

[21] Huang H, Pugsley MK, Fermini B, Curtis MJ, Koerner J, Accardi M, et al. Cardiac voltage-gated ion channels in safety pharmacology: Review of the landscape leading to the CiPA initiative. Journal of Pharmacological and Toxicological Methods. 2017;**87**:11-23

[22] Guidance for Industry Estimating the Maximum Safe Starting Dose in Initial Clinical Trials for Therapeutics in Adult Healthy Volunteers. Rockville, MD: Food and Drug Administration, Center for Drug Evaluation and Research (CDER); 2005

[23] Guideline on Strategies to Identify and Mitigate Risks for First-in-Human Clinical Trials with Investigational Medical Products. London, UK: European Medicines Agency; 2007. In: Agency EM, editor. London, UK; 2007

[24] Lutz RJ, Dedrick RL, Tuey D, Sipes IG, Anderson MW, Matthews HB. Comparison of the pharmacokinetics of several polychlorinated biphenyls in mouse, rat, dog, and monkey by means of a physiological pharmacokinetic model. Drug Metabolism and Disposition. 1984;**12**(5):527-535

[25] Offman E, Edginton AN. Contrasting toxicokinetic evaluations and interspecies pharmacokinetic scaling approaches for small molecules and biologics: Applicability to biosimilar development. Xenobiotica. 2013;**43**(6):561-569

[26] Gerlowski LE, Jain RK. Physiologically based pharmacokinetic modeling: Principles and applications. Journal of Pharmaceutical Sciences. 1983;**72**(10):1103-1127

[27] Fowler S, Morcos PN, Cleary Y, Martin-Facklam M, Parrott N, Gertz M, et al. Progress in prediction and interpretation of clinically relevant metabolic drug-drug interactions: A Minireview illustrating recent developments and current opportunities. Current Pharmacology Reports. 2017;**3**(1):36-49

[28] Safety testing of drug metabolites, guidance for industry. In: (CDER) FaDACfDEaR, editor. Rockville, MD: Food and Drug Administration Center for Drug Evaluation and Research (CDER); 2016

[29] Nakanishi T, Tamai I. Interaction of drug or food with drug transporters in intestine and liver. Current Drug Metabolism. 2015;**16**(9):753-764

[30] Hansen AR, Graham DM, Pond GR, Siu LL. Phase 1 trial design: Is 3+3 the best? Cancer Control. 2014;**21**(3):200-208

[31] Ludden TM. Nonlinear pharmacokinetics: Clinical implications. Clinical Pharmacokinetics. 1991;**20**(6):429-446

[32] Maganti L, Panebianco DL, Maes AL. Evaluation of methods for estimating time to steady state with examples from phase 1 studies. The AAPS Journal. 2008;**10**(1):141-147

[33] Mahajan R, Gupta K. Adaptive design clinical trials: Methodology, challenges and prospect. Indian Journal of Pharmacology. 2010;**42**(4):201-207

[34] Abuhelwa AY, Williams DB, Upton RN, Foster DJ. Food, gastrointestinal pH, and models of oral drug absorption. European Journal of Pharmaceutics and Biopharmaceutics. 2017;**112**:234-248

[35] Edholm M, Gil Berglund E, Salmonson T. Regulatory aspects of pharmacokinetic profiling in special populations: A European perspective. Clinical Pharmacokinetics. 2008;**47**(11):693-701

[36] Guidance for Industry, Pharmacokinetics in Patients with Impaired Hepatic Function: Study Design, Data Analysis, and Impact on Dosing and Labeling. Rockville, MD: Food and Drug Administration, Center for Drug Evaluation and Research (CDER), Center for Biologics Evaluation and Research (CBER); 2003

[37] Guidance for Industry, Pharmacokinetics in Patients with Impaired Renal Function — Study Design, Data Analysis, and Impact on Dosing and Labeling. Revision 1 ed. Rockville, MD: Food and Drug Administration, Center for Drug Evaluation and Research (CDER); 2010

[38] Otagiri M. A molecular functional study on the interactions of drugs with plasma proteins. Drug Metabolism and Pharmacokinetics. 2005;**20**(5):309-323

[39] Drug Development and Drug Interactions: Table of Substrates, Inhibitors and Inducers Internet: Food and Drug Administration; 2017 [updated 2017 November 14; cited 2017

December 10]. Available from: https://www.fda.gov/drugs/developmentapprovalprocess/developmentresources/druginteractionslabeling/ucm093664.htm

[40] Yu J, Ritchie TK, Zhou Z, Ragueneau-Majlessi I. Key findings from preclinical and clinical drug interaction studies presented in new drug and biological license applications approved by the Food and Drug Administration in 2014. Drug Metabolism and Disposition. 2016;**44**(1):83-101

[41] Roffel AF, van Marle SP, van Lier JJ, Hartstra J, van Hoogdalem EJ. An evaluation of human ADME and mass balance studies using regular or low doses of radiocarbon. Journal of Labelled Compounds and Radiopharmaceuticals 2016;**59**(14):619-626

[42] Hinderling PH. Red blood cells: A neglected compartment in pharmacokinetics and pharmacodynamics. Pharmacological Reviews. 1997;**49**(3):279-295

Chapter 5

Hepatotoxicity by Drugs

Alejandra Cano Paniagua and Pedro Amariles

Additional information is available at the end of the chapter

http://dx.doi.org/10.5772/intechopen.72005

Abstract

Hepatotoxicity is the injury or liver damage caused by exposure to drugs; it is an adverse drug reaction that may be uncommon but serious. The hepatic injury can be classified into hepatocellular, cholestatic and mixed, caused by increase in alanine aminotransferase and alkaline phosphatase than upper limit of normal. The risk factors include idiosyncrasy, age, gender, alcohol consumption, concomitant use of other drugs, previous or underlying liver disease, genetic and environmental factors. Liver toxicity manifestations are generally accompanied by nonspecific symptoms such as abdominal pain, jaundice, fever, nausea, vomiting, diarrhea, pruritus and rash. Identification of hepatotoxicity is a complex process to perform; therefore, clinical scales have been developed, such as the Roussel Uclaf Causality Assessment Method (CIOMS/RUCAM) and the Clinical Diagnostic Scale (M & V CDS). Additionally, there is no specific treatment for hepatotoxicity, which is based on suspending the suspected drug and treating symptoms. The most commonly associated pharmacological groups are antibiotics, nonsteroidal anti-inflammatory analgesics (NSAIDs), antidepressants and anticonvulsants. Drug-induced liver injury has been an adverse event, hard to identify, prevent and treat; thereby, the pharmacist intervention can contribute to the diminution of the deleterious effects in patient health.

Keywords: drugs, hepatotoxicity, drug-induced liver injury, anti-infective agents, antineoplastic agents, pharmacist intervention

1. Introduction

The objective of this chapter is to explain hepatotoxicity by drugs and provide relevance to a health problem that can lead to death if neglected; even though there is published information about it, it is still limited in some parts of the world. On the other hand, it is intended to disclose some activities developed by a pharmacist in a case of one patient with hepatotoxicity by drugs, which can contribute to the improvement of a patient's health status by helping to identify and to prevent the cause of the problem. In addition, we present the key results obtained by a structured review made in PubMed/Medline using the terms such as "liver disease" and "drug-induced liver Injury", until December 2015, and articles available in English, Spanish and French that recognized any drug as a possible trigger of hepatotoxicity were selected. The information obtained in this structured review was analyzed and compiled to give a better understanding about hepatotoxicity.

Thereby, use of drugs had generated some noxious effects on patient's health; one of the organs that may be affected is the liver, because substances or its formed metabolites in the biotransformation process; drugs can induce liver injury. Hepatotoxicity is the injury or liver damage caused by exposure to drugs or other nonpharmacological agents [1]. It is an adverse drug reaction that may be uncommon but serious, and is the most common cause of drug withdrawal from the pharmaceutical market [2]. Hepatic toxicity incidence by drugs is variable, because several retrospective and prospective studies were reported [3].

There are two types of hepatotoxicity: intrinsic reaction which is dose-dependent and predictable (less common) and idiosyncratic reaction which is not dose-dependent and not predictable (more common). Besides, the hepatic injury can be classified into hepatocellular, cholestatic and mixed, caused by increase in alanine aminotransferase (ALT), that is, >2–3 times and/or increase in alkaline phosphatase (ALP), that is, >2 times the upper limit of normal [4, 5]. The risk factors include: idiosyncrasy, age, gender, alcohol consumption, smoking, concomitant use of other drugs, previous or underlying liver disease and genetic and environmental factors [6, 7]. Clinical and pathological manifestations of hepatotoxicity include acute and chronic hepatitis, fulminant hepatitis, cholestasis, ductopenia, granulomatous hepatitis and steatosis (steatohepatitis, macrovesicular or microvesicular steatosis) [6], generally accompanied by nonspecific symptoms such as abdominal pain, jaundice, fever, nausea, vomiting, diarrhea, pruritus and rash [8].

It is estimated that approximately 1100 drugs, excluding substances of abuse and natural products, are associated with hepatotoxicity reactions [9]. Although most lipophilic drugs may cause hepatic disorders, the most commonly associated pharmacological groups are antibiotics (amoxicillin-clavulanic acid and rifampicin), nonsteroidal anti-inflammatory analgesics (NSAIDs) (diclofenac and ibuprofen), antidepressants (paroxetine) and anticonvulsants (phenytoin, carbamazepine and valproic acid) [1, 10]. Identification of hepatotoxicity is a complex process to perform; therefore, in practice, this is based on considering the presence of such alteration, conducting a thorough investigation related to the use of any substance and ruling out other causes of liver disease [11]. In order to solve the difficulty of identification and to try to estimate the probability that a therapeutic agent is associated with a hepatic disease, clinical scales have been developed; there are scales such as the Roussel Uclaf Causality Assessment Method (CIOMS/RUCAM) and the Clinical Diagnostic Scale (M & V CDS) that assess factors such as absence or presence of confounding factors, temporal relation of hepatotoxicity with drug consumption, coexistence of risk factors, previous description in the literature, exclusion of other causes and effects of readministration of the drug [12]. In general, there is no specific treatment for hepatic toxicity by drugs, which is based on suspending the suspected drug, treating symptoms, avoiding other possible hepatotoxic agents and monitoring laboratory tests [13, 14].

The liver injury generated by hepatotoxic medicines has been an adverse event, hard to identify and prevent, because of the sensibility of each patient. There is no specific treatment, except with a few drugs, hence, it is not possible to guarantee the recovery of symptoms in all cases. In such a way, it is necessary to search strategies that allow optimization of the health care process of patients with hepatic toxicity. Thereby, the pharmacist intervention can contribute to the diminution of the deleterious effects in patient health, promoting the proper use of the drugs.

2. Drug-induced hepatotoxicity: an overview

Hepatotoxicity is defined as injury or liver damage caused by exposure to drugs or other nonpharmacological agents [1]. It is an adverse drug reaction that may be uncommon but serious, and therefore, have a considerable impact on health [2]. Hepatotoxicity generates between 1/600 and 1/3500 of all hospital admissions, 2–3% of hospitalizations for jaundice, 10% of acute jaundice hepatitis (being more than 40% in people over 50 years of age) and between 15 and 30% of cases of fulminant hepatic failure [15, 16]. In the United States, a multicenter prospective study showed that drugs, including acetaminophen, are the most common cause of acute liver failure, explaining 39% of cases and overcoming viral hepatitis A and B, which represent 12% [17]. On the other hand, in France, an incidence of 13.9 (±2.4) cases per 100,000 inhabitants is estimated, corresponding to an annual global frequency of 8.1 (±1.5) cases [18]. In Switzerland, the estimated incidence is 2.2 per 100,000 inhabitants over 15 years of age; while in Spain, the annual incidence of severe liver disease is estimated as 7.4 per 1,000,000 population (95% confidence interval between 6.0 and 8.8) [10]. There are some countries in which evidence about incidence of liver injury by drugs is limited [19], generally, published information is based on clinical case reports.

Although hepatotoxicity is less frequent than other adverse drug effects, due to its severity and is the most common cause of drug withdrawal in the pharmaceutical market, it is assessed as a major adverse event [20], so, it is a frequent impediment to the development of drugs by pharmaceutical companies. In the past 20 years, in Europe and the United States medications such as troglitazone, bromfenac, trovafloxacin, ebrotidine, nimesulide, nefazodone, ximelagatran, lumiracoxib, pemoline and tolcapone have been withdrawn from the market [10, 21–23]; currently, some of them are retired worldwide.

The identification of hepatotoxicity is a complex process to perform; therefore, in clinical practice, it is based on considering the presence of such alteration, investigate about the use of any substance and ruling out other causes of liver disease [19]. It is necessary to identify all drugs used (prescription and over-the-counter), natural products, food, exposure to industrial toxics or substance abuse; moreover, try to identify the offending agent and to search for a description in literature may help. Besides, the chronological relationship between exposure to the suspected agent and the hepatotoxic reaction is a key to define causality; the drugs used in the last 3 months should be considered as suspects. The presence of hypersensitivity manifestations (rash, fever and eosinophilia) improves identification process as well as histological analysis through liver biopsy [24]. When a re-exposure to the suspected agent appears, it becomes a very conclusive indicator of causality.

There is no specific treatment for hepatic toxicity by drugs, which is based on suspending the suspected drug, treating symptoms (use of corticosteroids for hypersensitivity reactions), avoiding other possible hepatotoxic agents and continuous monitoring of laboratory tests [13, 14]. There are some exceptions of antidotes for treating liver toxicity by certain drugs such as the use of N-acetyl cysteine as an antidote for acetaminophen toxicity, or N-acetyl cysteine itself for the treatment of hepatotoxicity by phenytoin and carbamazepine, or carnitine for valproic acid toxicity [25]. With the suspension of the offending drug, in most cases, the health of the patients tends to improve; however, in other cases, the damage continues to progress and hospitalization is necessary, when irreversible liver failure occurs, liver transplantation is required and if the liver tissue damage is severe, patients can die in a few hours.

3. Hepatotoxicity associated to drugs

3.1. Expression of hepatotoxicity

Hepatotoxicity induced by drugs or toxins can be grouped into two types: intrinsic reactions (less common) and idiosyncratic reactions (more common) [6, 7, 26]. Intrinsic reactions are predictable, dose-dependent and reproducible in animal models; injury is produced trough toxic metabolites of drugs such as free radicals (generating lipid peroxidation), electrophilic molecules (formation of covalent bonds with hepatic proteins) or active oxygen molecules (generating peroxidation as well). Idiosyncratic reactions are not predictable, not dose-dependent and not reproducible in animals; there are many drugs capable of causing this type of reaction [11, 27]. The underlying mechanism of the idiosyncratic reaction may be a genetic polymorphism of the cytochrome P450 (CYP450) system, responsible for the drugs hepatic biotransformation. There are two types of idiosyncratic reactions: immune (characterized by hypersensitivity-type reaction) and metabolic [7, 13] (related to metabolism of substances).

3.2. Mechanisms of hepatotoxicity

The hepatocytes, cholangiocytes, Kupffer cells, ductal and endothelial cells are involved in the mechanisms by which drugs cause hepatotoxicity [28]; having direct effects on cellular organelles such as mitochondria, endoplasmic reticulum, cytoskeleton, microtubules or nucleus.

The drug metabolites generated in the liver through biotransformation can cause hepatic damage because formation of toxic or reactive substances such as electrophilic chemicals or free radicals [29], and thus an unchain a variety of chemical reactions may happen. These mechanisms can either generate necrosis or apoptosis or both. The following are some of the main mechanisms of liver injury [30]:

- Mitochondrial dysfunction: may be generated by the disruption of β-oxidation of lipids and oxidative energy production within the hepatocytes. Mitochondrial membrane permeabilization can lead to apoptosis, a rupture in mitochondrial membrane can lead to ATP depletion and subsequent necrosis, and an abnormal function can also lead to fat accumulation, so steatosis can be present [31].

- Immune response: is attributed to the formation of new antigens, this give origin to the idiosyncratic hepatotoxicity. Moreover, it can be accompanied by presence of inflammatory cells such as neutrophils and lymphocytes.
- Oxidative stress: is produced by ATP depletion accompanied by increase in intracellular calcium concentration, it can generate necrosis [28].
- Lipid peroxidation: is generated by the interaction between free radicals and fatty acids in membrane, the subsequent reaction may produce electrophilic metabolites generating DNA damage [32].

3.3. Type of injury

Liver histology is the ideal tool to define the pattern of hepatic toxicity; however, in clinical practice, most hepatotoxic lesions are classified according to biochemical tests [16]. In this way, according to Council for International Organizations of Medical Sciences (CIOMS), liver injury is considered, if at least one of the main hepatic enzymes, such as alanine aminotransferase, aspartate aminotransferase (AST), alkaline phosphatase and total bilirubin (TB), increases by two times, the upper limit of normal (ULN) [33]. Besides, liver injury is classified into the following three types of lesions:

- Hepatocellular lesion is characterized by damage in hepatocytes, which is manifested by elevation in ALT is more than two times the ULN or a ratio (R) of ALT/ALP greater than or equal to five.
- Cholestatic lesion is presented in cholangiocytes when ALP increases more than two times the ULN or R greater than two.
- Mixed lesion is showed when ALT and ALP increases more than two times the ULN or R is between two and five [4, 34].

On the other hand, Hy's rule defines liver damage when ALT level increases more than or equal to three times the ULN accompanied by bilirubin elevation [5, 35] and with or without rise of APL levels.

3.4. Risk factors

The influence of sensibility or idiosyncrasy of each person is recognized as an important risk factor. In addition, there are some factors that increase the probability of occurrence of hepatotoxicity [36]:

- Age: the elderly population is mostly affected by toxicity of drugs because of physiological changes and polymedication [10]; however, with valproic acid, young population is the most affected.
- Gender: female patients are the most susceptible for toxicity of drugs because of biological differences and pharmacokinetics; moreover, sex-specific factors such as menopause, pregnancy and menstruation may have influence.
- Alcohol consumption: may increase the toxic potential of pharmacological agents [37].

- Concomitant administration of drugs or herbal remedies: becomes a risk factor because it increases the probability of drug interactions.
- Previous or underlying hepatic diseases: may increase the risk of hepatotoxic agents [38].
- Genetic factors: related with genetic polymorphism in cytochrome P450 can unchain a hepatic lesion.

3.5. Clinical manifestations

The mechanisms of drug-induced liver injury are related with the clinical manifestations. The main clinical-pathological manifestations of hepatotoxicity and its histological findings include [6, 24, 26, 39]

- Acute hepatitis: caused by a wide variety of drugs and characterized by parenchymal inflammation, necrosis and Kupffer cells in sinusoids, which include symptoms like malaise, asthenia, anorexia, jaundice can be present but not always [15].
- Chronic hepatitis: characterized by persistent biochemical abnormalities beyond 6 months; fibrosis or cirrhosis may be present.
- Fulminant hepatitis: also called acute liver failure may cause death and its manifestations are necrosis and microvesicular steatosis.
- Cholestatic hepatitis: manifested by mixed hepatocellular and cholestatic injury accompanied by inflammation.
- Cholestasis: caused by bile plugs; include symptoms like jaundice and pruritus is characterized by minimal inflammation.
- Vanishing bile duct syndrome: presented by a paucity of bile ducts; inflammation and cholestasis may appear.
- Granulomatous hepatitis: presence of granulomas in portal tracts or parenchymal, accompanied with inflammation.
- Steatohepatitis: is the presence of fat in hepatocytes accompanied by inflammation and fibrosis.
- Macrovesicular steatosis: characterized by the presence of medium- or large-sized fat droplets in the cytoplasm of hepatocytes.
- Microvesicular steatosis: characterized by the presence of small-sized fat droplets in the cytoplasm of hepatocytes.

Many drugs have a specific pattern of injury in the liver but in some cases, the same drug can generate different patterns in the patients, the patterns and the drugs that cause them are presented in **Table 1**.

Many of these manifestations are accompanied by unspecific symptoms like discomfort, fever, nausea, vomiting, abdominal pain, jaundice, dark urine, pale stools, pruritus, loss of weight or

http://dx.doi.org/10.5772/intechopen.72005

Clinical pattern	Drugs
Acute hepatitis	Acetaminophen, allopurinol, carbamazepine, diclofenac, phenytoin, ibuprofen, isoniazid, naproxen, metoprolol, piroxicam, pyrazinamide, valproic acid [2, 39, 40]
Chronic hepatitis	Methyldopa, isoniazid, phenytoin [40], amoxicillin-clavulanic acid, bentazepam and atorvastatin [26]
Fulminant hepatitis	Lamotrigine, nimesulide, isoniazid, clarithromycin [40]
Cholestatic hepatitis	Phenytoin, amoxicillin-clavulanate [39], carbamazepine, chlorpromazine [6, 15]
Cholestasis	Anabolic steroids [6, 39], estrogens, contraceptive steroids [2, 26]
Vanishing bile duct syndrome	Sulfonamides, beta-lactams [39], carbamazepine [2]
Granulomatous hepatitis	Allopurinol, aspirin, carbamazepine, chlorpromazine, diltiazem, hydralazine, nitrofurantoin, penicillin, phenylbutazone, phenytoin, pyrazinamide, quinidine, sulfasalazine [6, 26, 40]
Macrovesicular steatosis	glucocorticoids and methotrexate [26], steroids, nitrofurantoin, gold, methotrexate, ibuprofen, indomethacin, sulindac, metoprolol [6]
Microvesicular steatosis	tetracycline, valproic acid, zidovudine, minocycline [6, 9, 26]
Steatohepatitis	Amiodarone, tamoxifen [6, 9, 36]

Table 1. Clinical patterns caused by drugs.

appetite, besides, signs like hepatic encephalopathy or increase in hepatic enzyme levels, making the identification of liver toxicity difficult.

3.6. Hepatotoxic drugs

It is estimated that approximately 1100 drugs, excluding substances of abuse and natural products, are associated with hepatotoxicity reactions [9]. Although most lipophilic drugs may cause hepatic impairment, the most commonly associated pharmacological groups are antibiotics (amoxicillin-clavulanic acid and rifampicin), nonsteroidal anti-inflammatory analgesics (NSAIDs) (diclofenac and ibuprofen), antidepressants (paroxetine) and anticonvulsants (phenytoin, carbamazepine and valproic acid) [8, 10, 18, 19]. In addition, a recent study shows that among intravenous drugs, antibiotics and antineoplastic are the pharmacological groups most associated with hepatic toxicity [41].

A structured review in PubMed/Medline was made using the terms: "liver disease" and/or "drug-induced liver injury", until December 2015, and articles available in English, Spanish and French that recognized any drug as a possible trigger of hepatotoxicity were selected; this review excluded articles reporting hepatotoxicity related with other agents different to drugs, any liver disease, reports of clinical trials about predictive patterns of injury or studies of stem cells. Then, some information was extracted regarding: expression of hepatotoxicity, type of injury, mechanisms of hepatotoxicity, risk factors and clinical manifestations. To assess the probability of occurrence of hepatotoxicity and the type of injury, three categories were established: definite, probable and possible probability, according to evidence [42]. To report the results, a list was made with 181 drugs and 17 combined pharmaceutical forms or therapeutic regimen; these were selected as substances likely to develop hepatotoxicity. Eight drugs had definite probability: methotrexate, minocycline, vancomycin, everolimus, isoniazid, rifampicin, pyrazinamide and tamoxifen (**Table 2**). The drugs assessed as probable were 61 (**Table 3**) and as possible were 119 (**Table 4**) [43].

Drugs assessed as definite

Drug [code ATC]	**Hepatic toxcity expression**	**Lesion type (probability of occurrence)**	**Hepatic toxcity mechanism**	**Risk factors**	**Clinical and pathological manifestations**
Vancomycin [J01XA01]	Idiosyncratic (immunoallergic)	Hepatocellular (definite)	Direct toxicity or immune adverse reactions	Adult population	Increase of aminotransferases. Rash, fever, eosinophilia
Minocycline [J01AA08]	Idiosyncratic	Hepatocellular (definite)	Lipid peroxidation (necrosis)	Women from 16 to 57 years	Autoimmune hepatitis. Steatosis. Periportal inflammation, swelling and collapse hepatocytes, antinuclear antibody, eosinophilia. Increase of aminotransferases. Jaundice, fever, abdominal pain, rash, anorexia, nausea, arthralgia, fatigue, pruritus
Isoniazid, rifampicin, pyrazinamide [J04 AM05]	Idiosyncratic	Hepatocellular (probable)	Lipid peroxidation (necrosis). Formation of hepatotoxic metabolites	Genetic polymorphisms. Female, old age, VIH co-infection	Hepatic encephalopathy. Steatosis. Granulomatous inflammation, central necrosis. Increase of liver enzymes. Jaundice, abdominal pain, anorexia, nausea, dark urine, vomiting, asthenia
Tamoxifen [L02BA01]	Idiosyncratic	Hepatocellular (definite)	Disrupt of β-oxidation of lipids. Steatohepatitis	Women from 50 to 70 years. Overweight, hyperlipidemia, hypertension, diabetes, osteoporosis, alcohol consumption <20 g/day	Steatohepatitis. Fibrosis. Micronodular cirrhosis. Necrosis. Inflammatory infiltrate. Hepatomegaly, peliosis hepatis, increase in aminotransferases. Nausea, vomiting, malaise, right upper quadrant pain
Everolimus [L01XE10]	No information	No information	Possible direct toxicity or hepatotoxic metabolites	Neoplasms, liver transplantation	Increase of aminotransferases, fatigue
Methotrexate [L04AX03]	No information	Hepatocellular (possible)	Direct toxicity. Lipid peroxidation (necrosis). Dysfunction mitochondrial	Previous hepatic disease. Alcoholism, obesity, diabetes. Cumulative dose. Use of steroids. Previous exposure to hepatotoxins	Steatohepatitis. Fibrosis, cirrhosis. Inflammatory infiltrate. Necrosis. Increase of liver enzymes

Table 2. Drugs assessed as definite.

http://dx.doi.org/10.5772/intechopen.72005

Drugs assesses as probable			
Acarbose	Propylthiouracil	Diclofenac	Flutamide
Troglitazone	Methylprednisolone	Lumiracoxib	Etopóside
Papaverine	Doxapram hydrochloride	Nimesulide	Imatinib
Vitamin A	Benzarone	Sodium aurothiomalate	Ipilimumab
Amiodarone	Fluconazole	Allopurinol	Oxaliplatin
Propafenone	Itraconazole	Dantrolene	Temozolomide
Metildopa	Ketoconazole	Cyproterone acetate	Tioguanine
Perhexiline	Rifampicin	Halothane	Glatiramer
Enalapril	Efavirenz	Isoflurane	Azathioprine
Atorvastatin	Nevirapine	Bentazepam	Infliximab
Ezetimibe	Paracetamol	Lamotrigine	Buprenorphine
Flupirtine	Telithromycin	Valproic acid	Clometiazol
Nitrofurantoin	Ciprofloxacin	Tolcapone	Carbamazepine
Ornidazole	Trovafloxacin	Dextropropoxyphene	
Flucloxacillin			

Table 3. Drugs assessed as probable.

Drugs assessed as possible			
Ranitidine	Carmustine	Zolmitriptan	Amphotericin B
Glibenclamide	Cyclophosphamide	Enflurane	Clindamycin
Gliclazide	Cytarabine	Methoxyflurane	Dapsone
Glimepiride	Dacarbazine	Propofol	Fosfomycin
Metformin	Mitoxantrone	Sevoflurane	Sulfadimethoxine
Pioglitazone	Trabectedin	Thiopental	Amoxicillin
Rosiglitazone	Leflunomide	Imipramine	Nafcillin
Mesalamine	Sirolimus	Mirtazapine	Oxacillin
Mesalazine	Thalidomide	Nefazodone	Cefdinir
Sulfasalazine	Tocilizumab	Nomifensine	Erythromycin
Oxymetholone	Alfuzosin	Sertraline	Spiramycin
Esomeprazole	Tamsulosine	Felbamate	Doxycicline
Orlistat	Cyclofenil	Phenytoin	Levofloxacin
Thioctic acid nilutamide	Raloxifene	Phenobarbital	Daptomycin
Actinomycine D	Testosterone	Clozapine	Brivudin
Busulfan	Disulfiram	Quetiapine	Didanosine
Donepezil	Simvastatin	Risperidone	Zidovudine
Indicine N-oxide	Pravastatin	Methylphenidate	Atomoxetine
Loratadine	Naftidrofuryl	Amodiaquiea	Spironolactone
Octreoctide	Piroxicam	Mefloquine	Fosinopril
Ibuprofen	Rofecoxib	Quinine	Lisinopril
Oxaprozin	Aurothioglucose	Etretinate	Bromfenac
Indomethacin	Glucosamine	Alendronate	Acetylsalicylic acid
Terbinafine	Nicotinic acid	Methimazole	Pazopanib
Ajmaline	Labetalol	Dabigatran	Nafamostat
Quinidine	Nicardipine	Clopidogrel	Dipirone
Hydralazine	Diltiazem	Dalteparin	Mebendazole
Candesartan	Tienilic acid	Phenprocoumon	Metronidazole
Irbesartan	Ferrous fumarate	Bosentan	
	Ticlopidine	Sitaxentan	

Table 4. Drugs assessed as possible.

4. Probability and causality assessment of drug-induced hepatotoxicity: scales and proposals

To solve the difficulty of identification of hepatotoxicity and to try to estimate the probability that a therapeutic agent is associated with a hepatic injury, clinical scales have been developed; these assess aspects such as absence or presence of confounding factors, temporal relation of hepatotoxicity with drug consumption, coexistence of risk factors, previous description in the literature, exclusion of other causes and effects of readministration of the drug. According to the score obtained, a range of causal probability is established.

In this sense, there are scales, such as the Roussel Uclaf Causality Assessment Method scale (RUCAM) and the Clinical Diagnostic Scale (M&V CDS), considering that the RUCAM scale is more appropriate than M&V CDS [12], besides, facilitates to distinguish when patient is using concomitants drugs. However, despite their theoretical utility and being validated, these scales are hardly used in clinical practice [22]. To promote its use, it is advisable to have knowledge of the possible agents associated with hepatotoxicity and to reduce subjectivity bias at the time of its application.

5. Hepatotoxic medicines during pregnancy

Twelve hepatotoxic agents were identified as drugs with probability to cause injury in pregnant women are as follows: acetaminophen, alpha-methyldopa, labetalol, methotrexate, saquinavir, nevirapine, propylthiouracil, methimazole, carbimazole, nitrofurantoin, acetylsalicylic acid and piperidolate. Some characteristics associated with these drugs were the time of reaction onset, weeks of pregnancy (between 3 and 36 weeks), risk factors (age and chronic diseases), clinical manifestations (elevation of transaminases, pruritus, vomiting, anorexia and jaundice) and outcomes (liver transplantation and death of mother and/or fetus). In this sense, pregnant women between the second and third decade of age may have an increased risk of liver problems due to the use of medications such as methotrexate, alpha-methyldopa and propylthiouracil. For drugs such as acetaminophen, acetylsalicylic acid, piperidolate, nitrofurantoin, methotrexate and alpha-methyldopa, information about frequency of hepatotoxic reactions during gestation is limited, whereas for antithyroid drugs, the frequency of occurrence of hepatotoxicity can be found between 0.1 and 0.2% of the pregnant population using these drugs [44]. The management in cases of hepatotoxicity in pregnant women must be the suspension of the offending drug, which in most cases afford to improve the symptomatology and prevent fatal outcomes.

6. Pharmacist and prevention of drug-induced hepatotoxicity

Currently, there is a need to discuss about interdisciplinary groups to provide comprehensive patient care; and the pharmacist is a part of this. Through knowledge of the important aspects of hepatotoxicity (hepatotoxic drugs, symptoms, risk factors, pathological antecedents and patient habits), it is possible for pharmacist to carry out prevention activities and promote the proper use of medications, decreasing deleterious effects on health of patient. Besides, feedback in the interdisciplinary group may optimize the reaction time in a liver injury case.

Identification of liver toxicity is difficult, because it has no specific manifestations; however, having in mind, this health problem may contribute to a fast clinical response. The next actions may help to identify drug-induced liver toxicity:

- In the blood samples, analyze if an alteration of liver tests is present: increase in alanine aminotransferase more than three times and/or increase in alkaline phosphatase more than two times the upper limit of normal.
- Ask treating physician or nurse about pathological antecedents like acute coronary syndrome, autoimmune diseases, previous or underlying liver disease or liver tumors, viral hepatitis, alcohol or substances abuse and blood transfusion, to rule out other causes of liver test alterations.
- Interview the patient or companion and ask about symptoms like abdominal pain, fever, nausea, vomiting, jaundice, dark urine, pale stools, asthenia, loss of weight or appetite; risk factors such as concomitant administration of drugs or herbal remedies, alcohol consumption, pregnancy or tattoos, use of medications at home and self-medication. Besides, it is important to know about the suspected drug, the beginning or cessation time, dose, frequency of use and route of administration.
- To know about the drugs used by the patient; it is recommended to search about adverse reactions in published information.
- Use a causality assessment of drug-induced liver injury scale like RUCAM, to define the causing agent, as propose in **Diagram 1**.

To prevent death or harmful effects, it is necessary to suspend the hepatotoxic drug, monitoring liver test and use other medications such as N-acetylcysteine or corticosteroids (prednisone, prednisolone and betamethasone) to improve the status of patient health [36]. Also, it is important to educate patient in proper use of drugs to prevent the occurrence of hepatotoxicity.

7. Comments and conclusions

Many drugs are hepatotoxic agents, most of these drugs generate idiosyncratic reactions and cause hepatocellular damage in a wide range of patients in different age groups; and moreover, concomitant medications may deteriorate the clinical features of patients. Elevation of liver enzymes, fever and jaundice are common signs and symptoms, with identification and suspension of offending drug, patients present an adequate evolution.

On the other hand, it is important to have in mind that some patients are asymptomatic and the liver injury identification is based only on the elevation of liver enzymes; therefore, monitoring of liver tests is important to prevent serious effects. In addition, knowing the risk factors and habits of patient can improve the response time in a possible case.

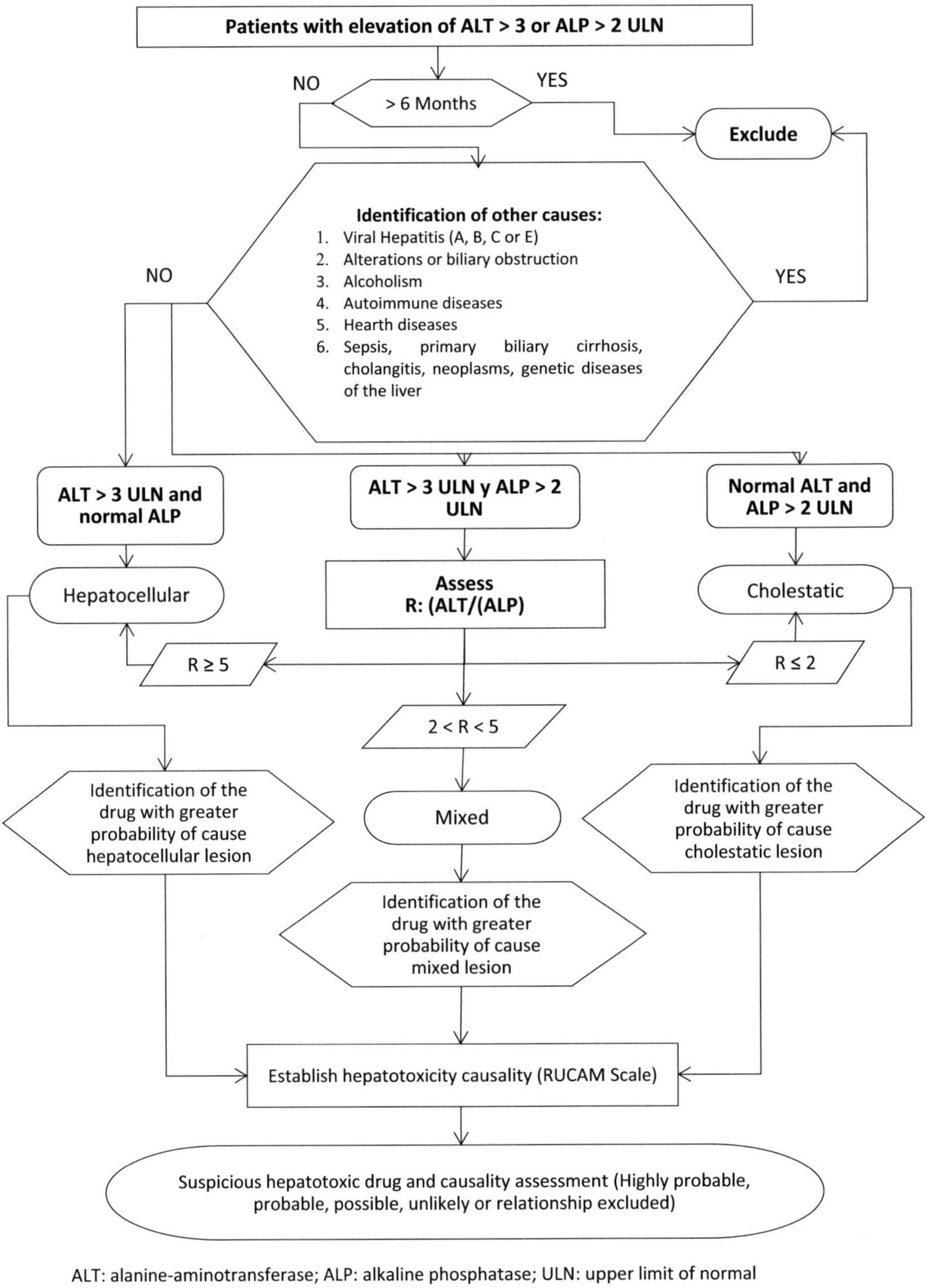

Diagram 1. Identification of hepatotoxicity.

It is advisable to use RUCAM scale to obtain a correct judgment when the probability of hepatotoxicity or any doubt exists. While there are other scales present, RUCAM allows discern when confusing factors or concomitant drugs are present.

Author details

Alejandra Cano Paniagua and Pedro Amariles*

*Address all correspondence to: pedro.amariles@udea.edu.co

Research Group on Pharmaceutical Prevention and Promotion, University of Antioquia, Medellin, Colombia

References

[1] Tejada F. Hepatotoxicidad por Fármacos. Revista Clínica de Medicina de Familia. 2010;**3**(3):177-191

[2] Andrade R, Robles M, Fernández-Castañer A, López-Ortega S, López-Vega M-C, Lucena M-I. Assessment of drug-induced hepatotoxicity in clinical practice: A challenge for gastroenterologists. World Journal of Gastroenterology. 2007;**13**(3):329-340

[3] Bell LN, Chalasani N. Epidemiology of idiosyncratic drug-induced liver injury. Seminars in Liver Disease. 2009;**29**(4):337-347

[4] Danan G, Benichou C. Causality assessment of adverse reactions to drugs-I. A novel method based on the conclusions of international consensus meetings: Application to drug-induced liver injuries. Journal of Clinical Epidemiology. 1993;**46**(11):1323-1330

[5] Reuben A. Hy's Law. Hepatology. 2004;**39**(2):574-578

[6] Ramachandran R, Kakar S. Histological patterns in drug-induced liver disease. Journal of Clinical Pathology. 2009;**62**:481-492

[7] Fisher K, Vuppalanchi R, Saxena R. Drug-induced liver injury. Archives of Pathology & Laboratory Medicine. 2015;**139**:876-887

[8] Martí L, Olmo J, Tosca J, Ornia E, Serra M, Rodríguez F, et al. Clinical evaluation of drug-induced hepatitis. Revista Espanola De Enfermedades Digestivas. 2005;**97**(4):258-265

[9] García-Cortés M, Andrade R, Lucena M, González-Grande R, Camargo R, Fernández-Bonilla E, et al. Hepatotoxicidad secundaria a fármacos de uso común. Gastroenterología y Hepatología. 2005;**28**(8):461-472

[10] Ibáñez L, Pérez E, Vidal X, Laporte J. Prospective surveillance of acute serious liver disease unrelated to infectious, obstructive, or metabolic diseases: Epidemiological and clinical features, and exposure to drugs. Journal of Hepatology. 2002;**37**(5):592-600

[11] Lee WM. Drug induced hepatotoxicity. The New England Journal of Medicine. 1995;**333**: 1118-1127

[12] Lucena M, Camargo R, Andrade R, Perez-Sanchez C, Sanchez De La Cuesta F. Comparison of two clinical scales for causality assessment in hepatotoxicity. Hepatology. 2001;**33** (1):123-130

[13] Adams D, Ju C, Ramaiah S, Uetrecht J, Jaeschke H. Mechanisms of immune-mediated liver injury. Toxicological Sciences. 2010;**115**(2):307-321

[14] Andrade R, López-Ortega S. Hepatitis Tóxicas. Revista Espanola De Enfermedades Digestivas. 2006;**98**(9):701

[15] Andrade R, Lucena M, González R. Hepatitis inducida por tóxicos. Formas clínicas agudas. Tratamiento. GH Continuada. 2003;**2**(5):197-202

[16] Larrey D. Epidemiology and individual susceptibility to adverse drug reactions affecting the liver. Seminars in Liver Disease. 2002;**22**(2):145-155

[17] Ostapowicz G, Fontana RJ, Schiødt FV, Larson A, Davern TJ, Han SHB, et al. Results of a prospective study of acute liver failure at 17 tertiary care centers in the United States. Annals of Internal Medicine. 2002;**137**(12):947-954

[18] Sgro C, Clinard F, Ouazir K, Chanay H, Allard C, Guilleminet C, et al. Incidence of drug-induced hepatic injuries: A French population-based study. Hepatology. 2002;**36**(2):451-455

[19] Hernández N, Bessone F, Sánchez A, Di Pace M, Brahm J, Zapata R, et al. Profile of idiosyncratic drug induced liver injury in Latin America. An analysis of published reports. Annals of Hepatology. 2014;**13**(2):231-239

[20] Bakke O, Manochia M, De Abajo F, Kaitin K, Lasagna L. Drug safety discontinuations in the United Kingdom, the United States, and Spain from 1974 through 1993: A regulatory perspective. Clinical Pharmacology and Therapeutics. 1995;**58**(1):108-117

[21] Onakpoya I, Heneghan C, Aronson J. Post-marketing withdrawal of 462 medicinal products because of adverse drug reactions : A systematic review of the world literature. BMC Medicine. 2016;**14**(10):1-11

[22] Lucena M, García-Cortés M, Cueto R, Lopez-Duran J, Andrade R. Assessment of drug-induced liver injury in clinical practice. Fundamental & Clinical Pharmacology. 2008;**22** (2):141-158

[23] Gunawan B, Kaplowitz N. Clinical perspectives on xenobiotic-induced hepatotoxicity. Drug Metabolism Reviews. 2004;**36**(2):301-312

[24] Kleiner D, Chalasani N, Lee W, Fontana R, Bonkovsky H, Watkins P, et al. Hepatic histological findings in suspected drug-induced liver injury: Systematic evaluation and clinical associations. Hepatology. 2014;**59**:661-670

[25] Björnsson E. Hepatotoxicity associated with antiepileptic drugs. Acta Neurologica Scandinavica. 2008;**118**(5):281-290

[26] Zhang X, Ouyang J, Thung S. Histopathologic manifestations of drug-induced hepatotoxicity. Clinics in Liver Disease. 2013;**17**(4):547-564

[27] Castell J, Miñana M. Hepatitis inducida por tóxicos. Mecanismos de toxicidad y patrones de lesión. GH Continuada. 2003;**2**(5):190-196

[28] Grattagliano I, Bonfrate L, Diogo C, Wang H, Wang D, Portincasa P. Biochemical mechanisms in drug-induced liver injury: Certainties and doubts. World Journal of Gastroenterology. 2009;**15**(39):4865-4876

[29] Kaplowitz N. Drug-induced liver injury. Clinical infectious diseases. 2011;**38**(Suppl 2):44-48

[30] Cullen JM. Mechanistic classification of liver injury. Toxicologic Pathology. 2005;**33**(1):6-8

[31] Gu X, Manautou J. Molecular mechanisms underlying chemical liver injury. Expert Reviews in Molecular Medicine. 2013;**14**(e4):1-24

[32] Pessayre D, Mansouri A, Berson A, Fromenty B. Mitochondrial involvement in drug-induced liver injury. Adverse Drug Reactions, Handbook of Experimental Pharmacology. 2010:311-365

[33] Bénichou C. Criteria of drug-induced liver disorders Report of an International Consensus Meeting. Journal of Hepatology. 1990;**11**:272-276

[34] Sistanizad M, Peterson GM. Drug-induced liver injury in the Australian setting. Journal of Clinical Pharmacy and Therapeutics. 2013;**38**(2):115-120

[35] Bjornsson E. Drug-induced liver injury: Hy's rule revisited. Clinical Pharmacology and Therapeutics. 2006;**79**(6):521-528

[36] Giordano C, Zervos X. Clinical manifestations and treatment of drug-induced hepatotoxicity. Clinics in Liver Disease. 2013;**17**(4):565-573

[37] Fernández-Castañer A, García-Cortés M, Lucena M, Borraz Y, Peláez G, Costa J, et al. An analysis of the causes, characteristics, and consequences of reexposure to a drug or compound responsible for a hepatotoxicity event. Revista Española de Enfermedades Digestivas. 2008;**100**(5):278-284

[38] Lee W. Drug-induced hepatotoxicity. New England Journal of Medicine. 2003;**349**:474-485

[39] Hayashi P, Fontana R. Clinical features, diagnosis, and natural history of drug-induced liver injury. Seminars in Liver Disease. 2014;**34**(2):134-144

[40] Tarantino G, Di Minno M, Capone D. Drug-induced liver injury: Is it somehow foreseeable? World Journal of Gastroenterology. 2009;**15**(23):2817-2833

[41] Ghabril M, Fontana R, Rockey D, Gu J, Chalasani N. Drug induced liver injury caused by intramuscular administered medications: The Drug Induced Liver Injury Network (DILIN) experience. Journal of Clinical Gastroenterology. 2013;**47**(6):553-558

[42] Amariles P, Giraldo N, Faus M. Interacciones medicamentosas: Aproximación para establecer y evaluar su relevancia clínica. Medicina Clínica (Barcelona). 2007;**129**(1):27-35

[43] Cano A, Amariles P. Liver toxicity caused by drugs: A structure review. Rev Colomb Gastroenterol. Forthcoming in 2017;**32**(4)

[44] Cano A, Amariles PA. Structured review of hepatotoxic medicines during pregnancy. Revista Colombiana de Gastroenterología. 2017;**32**(1):35-43

Chapter 6

Side Effects of Glucocorticoids

Irmak Sayın Alan and Bahadır Alan

Additional information is available at the end of the chapter

http://dx.doi.org/10.5772/intechopen.72019

Abstract

Glucocorticoids represent the most important and frequently used class of drugs in the management of many inflammatory and immunologic conditions. Beside these beneficial effects, glucocorticoids are also associated with serious side effects. Cushing's syndrome, adrenal suppression, hyperglycemia, dyslipidemia, cardiovascular disease, osteoporosis, psychiatric disturbances, and immunosuppression are among the most important side effects of systemic glucocorticoids. These side effects are especially noticeable at high doses for prolonged periods. Even in low-dose therapy, glucocorticoids could lead to serious side effects. The underlying molecular mechanisms of side effects of glucocorticoids are complex, distinct, and frequently only partly understood. This comprehensive article reviews the current knowledge of the most important side effects of glucocorticoids from a clinical perspective.

Keywords: glucocorticoids, systemic, mechanisms of actions, therapeutic use, side effects

1. Introduction

The term "glucocorticoids" (GCs) represents both naturally secreted hormones by adrenal cortex and anti-inflammatory and immunosuppressive agents. Since the successful use of hydrocortisone (cortisol), the principal glucocorticoid of the human adrenal cortex, in the suppression of the clinical manifestations of rheumatoid arthritis, many synthetic compounds with glucocorticoid activity have been manufactured and tested [1]. The differences between pharmacologic effects of synthetic GCs (SGCs) result from structural variations of their basic steroid nucleus and its side groups. These structural variations may affect the bioavailability of SGCs. These include gastrointestinal or parenteral absorption, plasma half-life, and metabolism in the liver, fat, or target tissues—and their abilities to interact with the glucocorticoid receptor and to modulate the transcription of glucocorticoid—responsive genes [2]. Structural variations reduce the natural cross-reactivity of SGCs with the mineralocorticoid receptor (MR), eliminating the offending salt-retaining effect. In addition to these, some variations increase SGCs' water solubility for parenteral administration or decrease their water solubility to improve topical potency [3, 4]. The main SGCs used in clinical practice together with their relative biological potencies and their plasma and biological half-lives are listed in **Table 1**.

GCs are 21-carbon steroid hormones. The delta-4,3-keto-11-beta,17-alpha,21-trihydroxyl configuration is required for glucocorticoid activity and is present in all natural and synthetic GCs. Approximately 90% of endogenous cortisol in serum is bound to proteins, primarily corticosteroid-binding globulin (CBG) and albumin. Conversely synthetic GCs other than prednisolone either bind weakly to albumin or circulate as free steroids, because they have little or no affinity for CBG. The free form of the GCs can easily diffuse through the membrane and can bind with high affinity to intracytoplasmic glucocorticoid receptors. GCs perform most of their effects owing to specific, immanent distributed intracellular receptors. Binding of the GCs to this receptor creates a complex, which then translocates into the nucleus, where it can interact directly with specific DNA sequences (glucocorticoid-responsive elements [GREs]) and other transcription factors. GCs are metabolized in the liver. The kidney excretes 95% of the conjugated metabolites, and the remainder is lost in the gut. Exogenous GCs have the same metabolic processes as endogenous GCs. The half-lives of synthetic GCs are generally longer than that of cortisol, which is approximately 80 minutes [8–13]. The mechanisms of actions of GCs are shown in **Figure 1**.

Glucocorticoids	**Equivalent dose (mg)**	**Glucocorticoid potency**	**HPA suppression**	**Mineralocorticoid potency**	**Plasma half-life (min)**	**Biologic half-life (h)**
Short-acting						
Cortisol	20.0	1.0	1.0	1.0	90	8–12
Cortisone	25.0	0.8		0.8	80–118	8–12
Intermediate-acting						
Prednisone	5.0	4.0	4.0	0.3	60	18–36
Prednisolone	5.0	5.0		0.3	115–200	18–36
Triamcinolone	4.0	5.0	4.0	0	30	18–36
Methylprednisolone	4.0	5.0	4.0	0	180	18–36
Long-acting						
Dexamethasone	0.75	30	17	0	200	36–54
Betamethasone	0.6	25–40		0	300	36–54
Mineralocorticoids						
Fludrocortisone	2.0	10	12.0	250	200	18–36
Desoxycorticosterone acetate	0			20	70	

Table 1. Glucocorticoid equivalencies (adapted from [5–7]).

http://dx.doi.org/10.5772/intechopen.72019

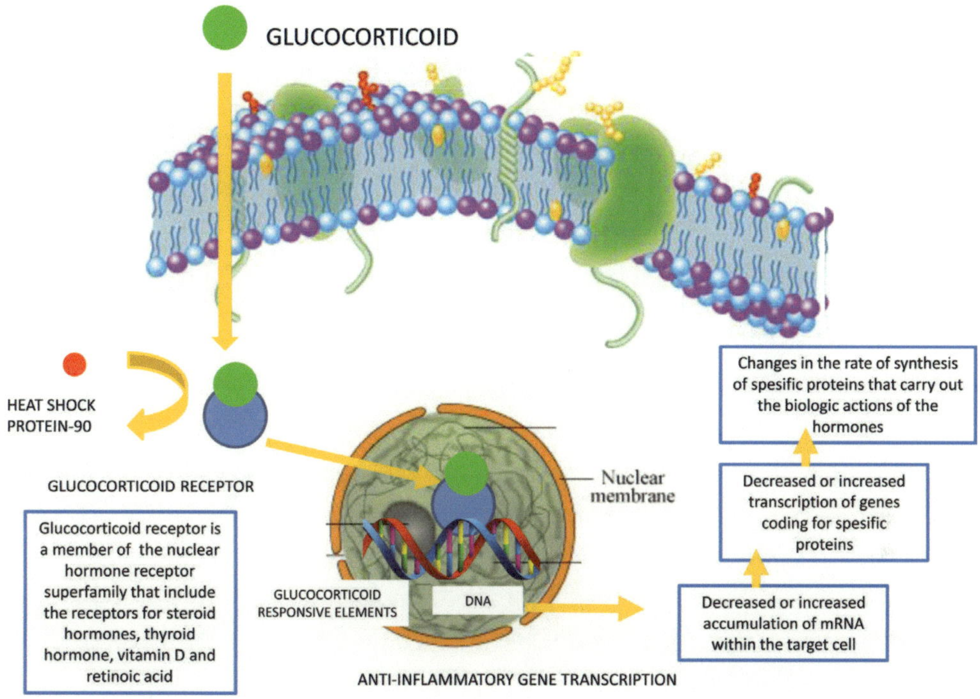

Figure 1. The mechanisms of actions of GCs.

GCs are used in nearly all medical specialties for systemic therapies. GCs represent the standard therapy for reducing inflammation and immune activation in asthma, as well as allergic, rheumatoid, collagen, vascular, hematological, neurological disorders, and inflammatory bowel diseases. Also GCs are used in renal, intestinal, liver, eye, and skin diseases and in the suppression of the host-vs.-graft or graft-vs.-host reactions following organ transplantation. SGCs administered as replacement therapy in primary or secondary adrenal insufficiency (AI), and as adrenal suppression therapy in glucocorticoid resistance and congenital adrenal hyperplasia. They are also used for some diagnostic purposes, such as in establishing Cushing's syndrome. Acute pharmacologic doses of GCs can be used in a small number of nonendocrine diseases, such as for patients suffering from acute traumatic spinal cord injury, with severe neurological deficits and bone pain even after surgery and critical illness-related cortisol insufficiency. In addition, all fetuses between 24 and 34 week gestation at risk of preterm delivery should be considered as candidates for antenatal treatment with GCs. Benefits of GCs have been showed in a number of other patients including high-risk cardiac surgery, liver failure, post-traumatic stress disorder, community acquired pneumonia, and weaning from mechanical ventilation [3, 4, 6, 7, 9, 14–18]. Common clinical uses of systemic GCs are shown in **Table 2**.

This comprehensive article aims to highlight the common side effects of systemic (oral and parenteral) GCs. First of all, the mechanisms of action of GCs will be described. Then the side effects of GCs will be discussed along with the pathophysiological mechanisms. While this section was being written, current literature and databases have been utilized.

Field of medicine	Disorder(s)
Allergy and respirology	• Moderate to severe asthma exacerbations
	• Acute exacerbations of chronic obstructive pulmonary disease
	• Allergic rhinitis
	• Atopic dermatitis
	• Urticaria/angioedema
	• Anaphylaxis
	• Food and drug allergies
	• Nasal polyps
	• Hypersensitivity pneumonitis
	• Sarcoidosis
	• Acute and chronic eosinophilic pneumonia
	• Interstitial lung disease
Dermatology	• Pemphigus vulgaris
	• Acute, severe contact dermatitis
Endocrinology	• Adrenal insufficiency
	• Congenital adrenal hyperplasia
Gastroenterology	• Ulcerative colitis
	• Crohn's disease
	• Autoimmune hepatitis
Hematology	• Lymphoma/leukemia
	• Hemolytic anemia
	• Idiopathic thrombocytopenic purpura
Rheumatology/immunology	• Rheumatoid arthritis
	• Systemic lupus erythematosus
	• Polymyalgia rheumatica
	• Polymyositis/dermatomyositis
	• Polyarteritis
	• Vasculitis
Ophthalmology	• Uveitis
	• Keratoconjunctivitis
Other	• Multiple sclerosis
	• Organ transplantation
	• Nephrotic syndrome
	• Chronic active hepatitis
	• Cerebral edema

Table 2. Common clinical uses of systemic GCs (adapted from [19]).

2. Mechanism of actions

GCs affect many, if not all, cells and tissues of the human body, thus awakening a wide variety of changes that involve several cell types concurrently [20].

2.1. Gene transcription

Binding of the receptor to GREs may cause either enhancement or suppression of transcription of responsive downstream genes. GCs inhibit the synthesis of almost all known inflammatory cytokines [21, 22].

2.2. Post-translational events

GCs also inhibit secretion and synthesis of inflammatory molecules (IL-1, IL-2, IL-6, IL-8, tumor necrosis factor, inflammatory eicosanoids, and cyclooxygenase-2) by affecting post-translational events [23].

2.3. Effect on the distribution of blood cells

The administration of glucocorticoids predictably results in neutrophilic leukocytosis, dramatic reductions in circulating eosinophils and basophils, transient minor reductions in monocytes and total lymphocytes. Acute lymphopenia normalizes by 24–48 hours. GCs have no direct effects on erythrocyte and platelet counts. But anemia and thrombocytosis can heal with improvement of chronic inflammation [24, 25].

3. Changes in cell function and survival

3.1. Neutrophils

The most important effect of GCs on neutrophils is the inhibition of neutrophil adhesion to endothelial cells. This effect reduces trapping of neutrophils in the inflamed region and probably is responsible for the characteristic hematological change—neutrophilia. GCs at pharmacologic doses, only modestly impair neutrophil functions, such as lysosomal enzyme release, the respiratory burst, and chemotaxis to the inflamed region. Lower doses do not affect these functions [26, 27].

3.2. Monocytes and macrophages

GCs antagonize macrophage differentiation and inhibit many of their functions. GCs (1) supress myelopoiesis and inhibit expression of class II major histocompatibility complex antigens induced by interferon-γ; (2) block the release of numerous cytokines, such as interleukin-1, interleukin-6, and tumor necrosis factor-α; (3) suppress production and release of pro-inflammatory prostaglandins (PGs) and leukotrienes; (4) suppress phagocytic and microbicidal activities of activated macrophages; (5) reduce the clearance of opsonized bacteria by the reticuloendothelial system; (6) reduce accumulation of monocytes and macrophages in the tissues [28–31].

3.3. Eosinophils, basophils, and mast cells

GCs support eosinophil apoptosis. In addition to this, GCs decrease the accumulation of eosinophils and mast cells to the allergic reaction sites. Also, GCs inhibit IgE-dependent release of histamine and leukotriene C4 from basophils, and they also inhibit degranulation both production of cytokines and degranulation of mast cells and eosinophils [26, 32, 33].

3.4. Natural killer cells (NKC)

Total numbers of circulating NKC are not significantly altered following administration of GCs. But, sustained upregulation of NKC activation genes were observed [34].

3.5. Endothelial cells

GCs have profound effects on the activation/function of endothelial cells and certainly inhibit vascular permeability. GCs inhibit directly the expression of adhesion molecules on both leukocytes and endothelial cells. GCs inhibit endothelial adhesion, as well as indirect effects due to the inhibition of transcription on cytokines (interleukin-1 and tumor necrosis factor) which upregulate endothelial adhesion molecule expression [25].

3.6. T lymphocytes

Administration of the GCs causes a dramatic diminution of in vitro antigen responsiveness of T lymphocytes. The generation, proliferation, and function of helper and suppressor T cells and cytotoxic T cell responses are inhibited by GCs. These effects are due to the inhibition of the release of certain cytokines. GCs also inhibit the acute generation of both T helper type 1- and T helper type 2-derived cytokines by activated T cells. But the inhibitory effect on expression of T helper type 1-derived cytokines is greater [35–38].

3.7. B lymphocytes and immunoglobulin levels

GCs have gradual effects on B cell activation, proliferation, and differentiation. B lymphocytes are relatively resistant to the immunosuppressive effects of GCs in contrast to T lymphocytes. Once B cells are activated, they differentiate into immunoglobulin-secreting plasma cells. But GCs have only minimal effects on this differentiation process. The most important effect of GCs on B lymphocytes relevant with immunoglobulin production and secretion. GCs also increase immunoglobulin catabolism. A short course of treatment with GCs causes an evident and permanent decrease in serum IgG. In contrast, immunoglobulin E (IgE) levels may increase. Whether GCs inhibit immunoglobulin gene expression is not known. Consequently, low-dose GCs inhibits leukocyte traffic and cellular immune responses. But to suppress the functions of leukocytes and the humoral immune response, higher doses of GCs are needed. This variability of drug response is also obvious among different patients and diseases [39–43].

3.8. Dendritic cells and antigen presentation

GCs causes a significant reduction in circulating dendritic cells. Dendritic are the major stimulants of naïve T cells by presenting antigens. As a result, GCs impair the development of immunity to first encountered antigens [44].

http://dx.doi.org/10.5772/intechopen.72019

3.9. Fibroblasts

At supraphysiological concentrations, GCs suppress proliferation of fibroblasts and growth factor-induced DNA synthesis and protein synthesis, including synthesis of collagen and glycosaminoglycan. Also GCs have been shown to interact with two mediators of fibroplasia; transforming growth factor-β and vascular endothelial growth factor. Furthermore GCs induce fibronectin messenger RNA transcription, inhibit interleukin-1, tumor necrosis factor-α-induced metalloproteinase synthesis, and arachidonic acid metabolite synthesis [20, 28, 45, 46].

3.10. Prostaglandins

Suppression of inflammatory prostaglandins (PGs) is a major factor in the anti-inflammatory action of the GCs. The suppression of phospholipase A2 activity with GCs is mediated by the activation of inhibitors of the enzyme itself or by inhibition of enzyme synthesis. The glucocorticoid-linked lipocortin/annexin family of proteins may be involved in this process. A second step in prostaglandin synthesis is the formation of prostaglandin H2 from arachidonic acid by enzymes called cyclooxygenases. The COX-2 gene and protein are strongly upregulated in endothelial cells, fibroblasts, and macrophages, and by mediators, such as endotoxin and interleukin-1. But GCs strongly suppress the expression of COX-2 induced by inflammatory stimuli. Later, D'Adamio et al. identified a glucocorticoid-induced leucine zipper (GILZ). GILZ is a member of the leucine zipper protein family which belongs to the transforming growth factor β-stimulated clone-22 family of transcription factors. GILZ inhibits inflammatory cytokine-induced expression of COX-2, by this way mediates the anti-inflammatory effects of GCs [47–53].

4. Side effects of systemic glucocorticoids

Toxicity of GCs is one of the most common causes of iatrogenic illness associated with chronic inflammatory disorders. The side effects of GCs have been known for decades. But the exact risk-benefit ratio is incomplete and/or inconsistent, because usually it is difficult to differentiate the effects of GCs from the effects of the underlying accompanying diseases, other comorbidities,

Onset early in therapy, essentially unavoidable

- Emotional lability
- Enhanced appetite, weight gain, or both
- Insomnia

Enhanced in patients with underlying risk factors or concomitant use of other drug

- Glucocorticoid-related acne
- Diabetes mellitus
- Hypertension
- Peptic ulcer disease

When supraphysiologic treatment is sustained

- Cushingoid appearance
- Hypothalmic-pituitary-adrenal suppression
- Impaired wound healing
- Myopathy
- Osteonecrosis
- Increased susceptibility to infections

Delayed and insidious, probably dependent on cumulative dose	
• Atherosclerosis	• Growth retardation
• Cataracts	• Osteoporosis
• Fatty liver	• Skin atrophy
Rare and unpredictable	
• Glaucoma	• Pseudotumor cerebri
• Pancreatitis	• Psychosis

Table 3. The most common and serious side effects of GCs (adapted from [56]).

or the other medications. GCs associated side effects are dependent on both the average dose and the duration of therapy. Overall, it can be stated that prolonged application is a high-risk factor, whereas total dose is of secondary importance. Even in low-dose therapy, GCs could lead to serious side effects. The severity ranges from more cosmetic aspects (e.g. teleangiectasia, hypertrichosis) to serious disabling and even life-threatening situations (e.g. gastric hemorrhage). Single or multiple side effects can occur [12, 54, 55]. The side effects of GCs are the major limiting factor for the use of these agents. An overview of the most common and serious side effects of GCs is summarized in **Table 3**.

5. Adrenal insufficiency (AI)

The most common cause of AI is the chronic administration of high doses of GCs. This is called iatrogenic or tertiary AI. Exogenous GCs causes a significant suppression of the hypothalamic-pituitary-adrenal axis (HPA) even in small doses for only few days. Consequently, the adrenal cortex loses the ability to produce cortisol in the absence of adrenocorticotrophic hormone (ACTH). When the suppression of ACTH levels prolonges, this situation causes atrophy of the adrenal cortex and secondary adrenal insufficiency. The use of systemic GCs results in higher systemic levels of corticosteroids than in cases of compartmental use, as a result leads to higher percentages of AI. Adrenal suppression is more likely in the following situations: **(1)** longer duration of treatment. The influence of smaller doses over longer durations is highly variable. After long-term systemic therapy with GCs (more than 1 year), AI has to be expected in 100% of the patients. **(2)** Supraphysiologic doses, stronger formulations, and longer acting formulations (**Table 4**). If the patients are taking doses of prednisone of ≥20 mg daily for ≥3 weeks, this situation should be considered as adrenal suppression. AI lasting for more than 4 weeks has been demonstrated after treatment with high-dose dexamethasone for 28 days [57–64].

Adrenal suppression is less likely in the following situations: (1) regimens that mimic the diurnal rhythm of cortisol (higher dose in the morning, lower dose in the afternoon) and (2) alternate-day dosing of steroids. The possible risk of this side effect is unknown. At the same time, individual responses to GCs may be highly different. The clinical presentation of AI is variable; many of the signs and symptoms are non-specific and can be mistaken for symptoms of intercurrent illness or the underlying condition being treated with GCs. Signs and symptoms of AI

Dose	Definition
Low dose	≤7.5 mg prednisone equivalent/day
Medium	>7.5 mg but ≤30 mg prednisone equivalent/day
High	>30 mg but ≤100 mg prednisone equivalent/day
Very high	>100 mg prednisone equivalent/day
Pulse therapy	≥250 mg prednisone equivalent/day for 1 day or a few days
Prednisone or prenisolone 5 mg≈/hydrocortisone 20 mg≈/dexamethasone 0.75 mg.	

Table 4. The supraphysiologic dosing and interconversion of SGCs (adapted from [66, 67, 69]).

Adrenal suppression	• Weakness/fatigue • Malaise • Nausea • Vomiting • Diarrhea • Abdominal pain • Headache (usually in the morning) • Fever • Anorexia/weight loss • Myalgia • Arthralgia • Psychiatric symptoms • Poor linear growth in children • Poor weight gain in children • Clinical signs of Cushing syndrome
Adrenal crisis	• Hypotension • Decreased consciousness • Lethargy • Unexplained hypoglycemia • Hyponatremia • Seizure • Coma

Table 5. Signs and symptoms of adrenal insufficiency and adrenal crisis (adapted from [72]).

and adrenal crisis are listed in **Table 5**. AI often occurs when the exogenous GCs are withdrawn too rapidly or, in the case of stressful conditions (e.g. surgery and infection), when higher levels of GCs may be required. In addition to AI and adrenal crisis decreased ACTH level related with the suppression of the HPA axis, leads to reduced general steroid-hormone production. This situation favors further side effects, such as hypogonadism and osteoporosis [55, 65–68].

5.1. Steroid withdrawal or adrenal insufficiency?

When GCs are tapered and their effects decline, patients might experience lethargy, myalgias, nausea, vomiting, and postural hypotension. In this situation, increasing the dose of GCs to prevent AI may delay recovery of the adrenal function. The treatment plan should be made by evaluating the risk/benefit ratio. At this point, patients may just need reassurance, symptomatic treatment, or if necessary, a brief (1-week) increase of the previous lowest dose, followed by reevaluation. Maximal caution is advised with any taper. Fortunately, the adrenal cortex repairs the ability to secrete sufficient amounts of cortisol for some period of time. Repair of endogenous cortisol secretion is expected after stopping the exogenous GCs. But the recovery time may vary among patients. The inhibition of the HPA axis function induced by exogenous GCs may persist for 6–12 months after treatment is withdrawn. In conclusion, all patients using GCs are at risk for AI. Clinicians should inform patients about the risk, signs, and symptoms of AI; and consider testing patients after cessation of high dose or long-term treatment with GCs [68].

6. Weight gain and lipodystrophy

GCs have reciprocal effects on adipose tissue metabolism, promoting both lipolysis and lipogenesis/adipogenesis, inducing irregularity of adipose tissue distribution (i.e. lipodystrophy). These effects are shown in **Figure 2** (adapted from [69]). About 60–70% of patients treated with GCs for a long-term period report weight gain. This is different from classical weight gain. A central hypertrophy of adipose tissue develops. Characteristic findings are facial adipose tissue (moon face), truncal obesity and dorsocervical adipose tissue (buffalo hump). In contrast, peripheral and subcutaneous adipose tissues get thinner. This specific changes are called Cushingoid features and related with lipodystrophy induced by GCs. Weight gain is the most common self-reported side effect. About two-thirds of patients exhibit Cushingoid features within the

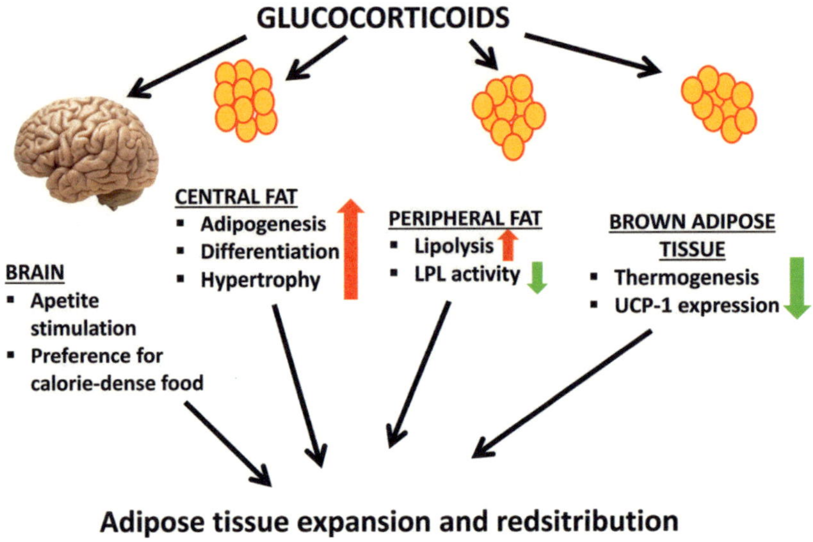

Figure 2. Mechanisms of glucocorticoid-induced weight gain and lipodystrophy.

first 2 months of therapy with GCs. These side effects are dependent on both the dose and duration of GCs. The risk of weight gain increases from the use of 5 to 7.5 mg per day of prednisone (or an equivalent). The risk of these side effects are higher in younger patients, females, those with a higher baseline body mass index, those with a higher initial caloric intake (>30 kcal/kg/day), and those with a baseline higher leptin and lower resistin levels. More importantly, these side effects are related with high blood pressure, blood glucose and triglyceride levels, and low high-density lipoprotein cholesterol levels (cardiovascular risk factors). Therefore, treatment with GCs increases the risk of coronary heart disease, cardiac insufficiency, and stroke [70–74].

7. Cardiovascular disease

GCs have complex, and often conflicting, influences on cardiovascular disease (CVD) and cardiovascular risk. Patients chronically using exogenous GCs are at higher risk of CVD, such as coronary artery disease, heart failure, and stroke. In patients with rheumatoid arthritis, chronic obstructive pulmonary disease, and other conditions who were exposed to chronic exogenous GCs, a case-control study found a dose-response relationship between daily glucocorticoid dose and the risk of heart failure. The risk of ischemic heart disease was also increased. Patients taking ≥7.5 mg of prednisone per day or the equivalent had a significantly higher mixed risk of myocardial infarction, angina, coronary revascularization, hospitalization for heart failure, transient ischemic attack, and stroke. Exposure to GCs within the preceding 6 months was related with increased cardiovascular risks. The risks were higher with continuous use than intermittent use. The relationship between cardiovascular risk and GCs is confounded by the underlying inflammatory disease (e.g. rheumatoid arthritis and systemic lupus erythematosus). Because of chronic inflammation and treatment with higher doses of GCs, chronic inflammatory conditions may further increase the incidence of CVD. This increased risk is cumulative and dose-dependent, is mainly observed during the first month of treatment and is reduced when treatment is interrupted. In patients with inflammatory arthritis, increased mortality from heart disease has been established. Moreover, an association between GCs and the risk for atrial fibrillation and flutter has been established by several studies. Pulse GCs are additionally related with CVD. Sudden death caused by pulse dose GCs has been reported. But this tends to occur in patients with underlying CVD. Therefore, patients with underlying severe cardiac and renal disease should be closely monitored during pulse therapy with GCs [75–78].

Cardiovascular side effects of GCs can be explained by two mechanisms: (1) direct influence on the function of the heart and vasculature and (2) increasing cardiovascular risk factors. Glucocorticoid receptor is known to be expressed in the heart. By this way GCs exert direct effects on cardiomyocytes. The interaction of GCs with the vascular wall is impaired in CVD. Some well-known cardiovascular risk factors, such as hypertension, insulin resistance, hyperglycemia, and dyslipidemia are more commonly observed in glucocorticoid exposed people. The main effects of GCs on cardiovascular risk are likely due to interaction with the kidney, liver, adipose tissue, and central nervous system. The effects of GCs on homeostasis are presumably due to renal sodium retention and intravascular volume overload. There is also evidence for additional, non-renal mechanisms. This confirms that GCs can interact directly with the cells of the heart and vascular wall. By this way, GCs may alter their function and structure. In patients with chronic inflammatory disease, carotid plaque and arterial distensibility (independent of cardiovascular risk factors and clinical manifestations) have been established. In patients with systemic lupus erythematosus administration of GCs decreased the effectiveness of pravastatin [79–83].

8. Hyperglycemia and diabetes

GCs are the most common cause of drug-induced hyperglycemia and diabetes. Hyperglycemia and diabetes induced by GCs, is defined as an abnormal increase in blood glucose associated with the use of GCs in a patient with or without a prior history of hyperglycemia or diabetes. GCs cause an exaggerated postprandial hyperglycemia and insensitivity to exogenous insulin. Thus, GCs have a greater effect on postprandial compared to fasting glucose. Postprandial hyperglycemia (defined as blood glucose 200 mg/dL 2 hours after a meal) is a much more sensitive indicator for hyperglycemia and diabetes induced by GCs. The exact prevalence is not known. The incidence of hyperglycemia and diabetes in hospitalized patients treated with GCs without a known history of diabetes is >50%. GCs increases by two- to fourfold the risk of hyperglycemia and diabetes in non-diabetic subjects. Treatment with exogenous GCs disrupts the glycemic balance of known diabetics [84–87].

Development of glucocorticoid-induced diabetes depends on the dose and duration of exposure. A study found that the risk for hyperglycemia increased substantially with increasing daily steroid dose. The risk may change with the type of the GCs, related with biochemical properties (e.g. potency of the anti-inflammatory and metabolic effects and duration of the effects). But, there is little difference between the GCs most frequently used (i.e. prednisone, prednisolone, and methylprednisolone). The effects of GCs on glucose excursions are observed within hours (6–8 hours) of exposure. The predisposing factors for hyperglycemia and diabetes induced by GCs have been suggested to be overweight, old age, non-white ethnicity, previous glucose intolerance, reduced sensitivity to insulin or impaired insulin secretion stimulated by glucose, female sex, Down syndrome, puberty, the severity of the disease itself, a family history of diabetes, type A30, B27, and Bw42 human leukocyte antigens (HLA); and receiving a kidney transplant from a deceased donor. Solid organ transplant patients treated with GCs, 10–20% of them develop diabetes, especially within the first months of exposure. Other immunosuppressive agents can also disrupt glycemic control through other mechanisms. Usually, hyperglycemia and diabetes induced by GCs improves with dose reductions and usually reverses when therapy is discontinued, but patients with high risk may develop persistent diabetes [88–91].

The pathophysiology of glucocorticoid-induced diabetes involves (1) increase in insulin resistance and (2) reduced glucose uptake in muscle and adipose tissue (via insulin-sensitive glucose transporter type 4) as a consequence GCs cause decreasing glucose uptake and glycogen synthesis. On the other hand GCs have profound and reciprocal effects on glyceroneogenesis in liver and adipose tissue. GCs increase the amount of fatty acids released into the blood. Increased fatty acids interfere with glucose utilization and causes insulin resistance, particularly in skeletal muscle. (3) Increased glucose production, increased hepatic gluconeogenesis via peroxisome proliferator-activated receptor α. (4) Direct effects on pancreatic β cells including inhibition of the production and secretion of insulin, a proapoptotic effect on β cells, a reduction in insulin

http://dx.doi.org/10.5772/intechopen.72019

biosynthesis, and β cell failure. (5) GCs may modulate the expression and activity of adipokines, such as adiponectin, leptin, and resistin. By this way GCs may disrupt insulin sensitivity and may also reduce the insulinotropic effects of glucagon-like peptide-1 [92–97].

9. Osteoporosis and osteonecrosis

9.1. Osteoporosis

GCs are the most common cause of secondary osteoporosis and nontraumatic osteonecrosis. GCs increase fracture risk in both adult men and women, regardless of bone mineral density (BMD) and prior fracture history. But fracture risk is related to the dose and duration of GCs, age, and body weight. Risk factors for osteoporosis induced by GCs are shown in **Table 6**. GCs cause significantly stronger losses of trabecular than of cortical bone. Fractures are most common in regions of the skeleton that are predominantly cancellous, such as the vertebral bodies and ribs. After discontinuation of GCs, fracture risk gradually declines to baseline over a year or two [98–100].

GCs induce osteoclastic activity initially (first 6–12 months), followed by a decrease in bone formation. GCs decrease bone formation by inhibiting osteoblastic activity in the bone marrow, suppressing osteoblast function, decreasing osteoblast life span, and promoting the apoptosis of osteoblasts and osteocytes. The effect of GCs on bone turnover is complex and can be divided into two groups (**Table 7**) [101–103].

Risk factor	Explanation
Advancing age	Elderly patients receiving glucocorticoid therapy have a 26-fold higher risk of vertebral fractures than younger patients and a shorter interval between initiation of treatment and the occurrence of fracture
Low body mass index	Significant risk factor for GIO and probably fractures as well
Underlying disease	Rheumatoid arthritis, polymyalgia rheumatica, inflammatory bowel disease, chronic pulmonary disease, and transplantation are independent risk factors
Family history of hip fracture, prevalent fractures, smoking, excessive alcohol consumption, frequent falls	All are independent risk factors for osteoporosis but have not been well studied in patients receiving glucocorticoids
Glucocorticoid receptor genotype	Individual glucocorticoid sensitivity may be regulated by polymorphisms in the glucocorticoid receptor gene
11β-HSD isoenzymes	11β-HSD1 expression increases with aging and glucocorticoid administration and thereby enhances glucocorticoid activation
Glucocorticoid dose (peak, current, or cumulative, duration of therapy, interval)	There may be no safe dose, although this is somewhat controversial. However, the risk of fracture unarguably escalates with increased doses and duration of therapy. Alternate day or inhalation therapy does not spare the skeleton
Low BMD	Glucocorticoid-induced fractures occur independently of a decline in bone mass but patients with very low bone density may be at higher risk

11β-HSD, 11β-hydroxysteroid dehydrogenase; BMD, bone mineral density.

Table 6. Risk factors for glucocorticoid-induced osteoporosis (adapted from [99]).

Direct effects	Indirect effects
1. Decreased bone formation	1. Decrease in net intestinal Ca^{2+} absorbtion
• Inhibition of osteoblasts replication	2. Inhibition of renal Ca^{2+} re-absorbtion
• Inhibition of osteoblastic apoptosis	3. Stimulation of parathyroid hormone secretion
• Inhibition of bone matrix synthesis	4. Inhibition of growth hormone secretion
2. Increased bone reabsorbtion	
• Stimulation of osteoclast synthesis	

Table 7. Effects of glucocorticoids on bone metabolism (adapted from [103]).

1. Dose and duration of therapy
2. Intra-articular administration
3. Polymorphisms in VEGF, GR, 11β-HSD2, COL2A1, PAI1, P-glycoprotein
4. Underlying disorders: renal insufficiency, transplantation, graft vs. host disease, inflammatory bowel disease, HIV, acute lymphoblastic leukemia, excessive alcohol intake, hypercoagulable states, sickle cell disease, radiation exposure
5. Dexamethasone causes greater skeletal complications than prednisone
VEGF: vascular endothelial growth factor; GR: glucocorticoid receptor; 11β-HSD2: 11β-hydroxysteroid dehydrogenase type2; COL2A1: collagen type II; PA1: plasminogen activator inhibitor 1; HIV: human immunodeficiency virus.

Table 8. Risk factors for glucocorticoid-induced osteonecrosis (adapted from [99]).

9.2. Osteonecrosis

The most common joint involved is the hip and GCs are the second most common cause. The incidence of osteonecrosis induced by GCs increase with higher doses and prolonged treatment. But can be seen with short-term exposure to high doses, and without osteoporosis. Osteonecrosis develops in 9–40% of adult patients receiving long-term GCs. Risk factors are shown in **Table 8** [104–106].

10. Hypertension

Glucocorticoid-induced elevation in blood pressure is classified as secondary hypertension and is a major risk factor for cardiovascular diseases. Blood pressure in humans is subjected to tight control by several physiologic systems that have pleiotropic effects and interact together in a complex fashion. GCs can cause hypertension by influencing these systems in different ways. One possible mechanism is the in vitro affinity of the non-selective mineralocorticoid receptor (MR) for the GCs. As a result, stimulation of the MR by exogenous GCs leads to renal Na^+ retention, volume expansion, and finally to an increase in blood pressure. Vascular tone (imbalance between vasoconstriction and vasodilation), centrally mediated mechanisms, renin-angiotensin system activation, cardiac hypercontractility, and endothelial cell dysfunction may also play a role. Enhanced reactive oxygen species and reduced nitric oxide (NO) bioavailability are the most important factors for endothelial cell dysfunction. The risk of hypertension is 2.2 times higher in patients treated with GCs, whatever the duration of exposure. The risk seems to increase with duration of exposure and daily dosage. A family history of essential hypertension may also predispose hypertension induced by GCs. People with glucocorticoid-induced lipodystrophy are at higher risk [107–110].

11. Dyslipidemia

GCs have a very important role in energy homeostasis and on lipid metabolism. Chronic exposure to exogenous GCs is a secondary cause of dyslipidemia. But the degree of lipid abnormalities in different clinical conditions is quite variable. These variabilities are related with the heterogeneity of the populations treated in terms of age, sex, underlying condition, glucocorticoid dose, and concomitant medications. All possible changes in lipid profile (i.e. isolated increase of triglyceride levels, increase of both cholesterol and triglycerides levels, absence of changes in lipid parameters, and improvement in lipid profile with increased HDL cholesterol) have been reported, excluding organ transplant recipients. Because transplanted patients concomitantly treated with other immunosuppressive drugs with side effects on the lipid metabolism (e.g. cyclosporine), which is a confounding factor. People with glucocorticoid-induced lipodystrophy are more likely to develop an unfavorable lipid profile. But interestingly, findings from the Third National Health and Nutrition Examination Survey suggest that GCs may have a beneficial effect on lipid profile in adults ≥60 years of age. GCs stimulate lipolysis and modulate free fatty acid (FFA) mobilization through various mechanisms. These mechanisms are summarized in **Figure 2**. Stimulation of lipolysis depends on dose and duration. Therefore in patients treated with GCs at high doses or for prolonged periods, regular monitoring of lipid profile is recommended [111–114] (**Figure 3**).

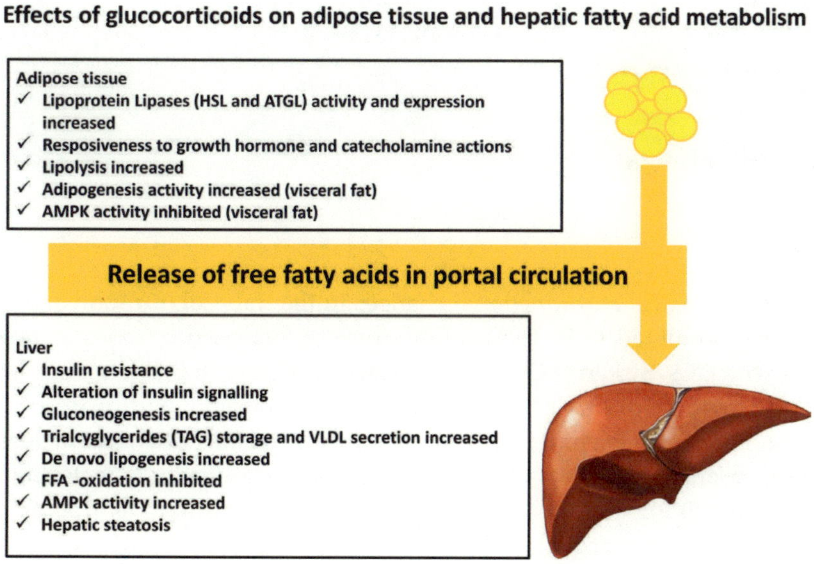

Figure 3. Effects of glucocorticoids on adipose tissue and hepatic fatty acid metabolism (adapted from [115]).

12. Gastrointestinal side effects

Side effects of GCs on the gastrointestinal system include peptic ulcers (PU), upper gastrointestinal bleeding (UGB), and pancreatitis.

12.1. PU

There is conflicting evidence related with the risk of PU for patients treated with glucocorticoid monotherapy. In a case-control study, there was no increased risk of PU at any dose or duration of glucocorticoid monotherapy. But in the same study, the combination of GCs with nonsteroidal anti-inflammatory drugs (NSAID), there was a significantly increased risk of peptic ulcer. Treatment with GCs may cause gastric irritation, more than PU [116, 117].

12.2. UGB

The incidence of UGB is low in patients treated with GCs alone and without a prior history of bleeding, but notably higher in patients receiving concomitantly anticoagulants and NSAIDs, and those with a history of bleeding. In the presence of different underlying diseases, such as rheumatoid arthritis, treatment with GCs may represent a more important risk factor for gastrointestinal complications than NSAIDs. In animal studies, GCs have been shown to increase gastric acid secretion, to reduce gastric mucus, to cause gastrin and parietal cell hyperplasia, and to delay the healing of ulcers [118–120].

12.3. Pancreatitis

Although the exact mechanism is unknown, incidence of GCs induced pancreatitis is well established in the medical literature. One case-control study showed that the risk of acute pancreatitis was increased among current users of oral GCs compared with nonusers. This risk was highest 4–14 days after drug dispensation and the risk gradually decreased thereafter. Pancreatitis, commonly reported in chronic exposure to GCs, especially in large doses for a wide variety of diseases [121].

13. Ocular side effects

13.1. Glaucoma

GCs induce morphological and functional changes in the trabecular meshwork (TM). These mechanisms are considered to be the leading cause of increased intraocular pressure during treatment with GCs. Systemic GCs are associated with a high incidence of glaucoma. All doses of GCs increase the risk for glaucoma. Nevertheless, doses of hydrocortisone 40 mg per day (prednisone 10 mg equivalent) were associated with an almost twofold increased risk. In patients over 40 years of age and with certain systemic diseases (e.g. diabetes mellitus, high myopia, connective tissue disease particularly rheumatoid arthritis), as well as relatives of patients with primary open-angle glaucoma (POAG), the risk for glaucoma induced by GCs increases. Glaucoma may lead to increased intraocular pressure, optic disc cupping, severe optic nerve damage, but considered a *silent* disease. *Because* there are no evident *symptoms* until visual loss. Discontinuation of GCs leads to reversal of intraocular hypertension within a few weeks, but the optic nerve damage is often permanent [122, 123].

13.2. Cataracts

Posterior subcapsular cataracts (PSC) induced by GCs appears bilaterally and is distinguishable from the more common types of cataract. Increased glucose levels, caused by an increased gluconeogenesis rate; inhibition of Na^+/K^+-ATPase; increased cation permeability; inhibition of glucose-6-phosphate-dehydrogenase; inhibition of RNA synthesis; loss of ATP; and covalent binding of steroids to lens proteins are the possible mechanisms. These changes are specific for PSC induced by GCs. The risk appears to be both duration and dose-dependent. PSC is more likely to occur at higher doses of GCs. But as with other side effects, lower doses (<5 mg prednisone per day) have been linked to PSC [123, 124].

13.3. Central serous chorioretinopathy (CSCR)

CSCR is also associated with systemic GCs. Symptoms are central visual blur and reduced visual acuity. GCs should be used cautiously in patients with a history of CSCR [125].

Exophthalmos and chorioretinopathy rarely occur. Consequently, before treatment with GCs, clinicians should ask about the history of glaucoma, cataracts, and CSCR; and patients with risk factors should be referred to ophthalmologic examination.

14. Immunosuppression and risk of infection

There are multiple anti-inflammatory and immunosuppressive effects of GCs (**Table 9**) [126]. These mechanisms may predispose patients to infections. The overall risk of infections is 50–60% higher in the patients exposed to GCs. The risk of infections can be related with dose and duration of GCs. Infection rates were not increased in patients given a daily dose of <10 mg or a cumulative dose of <700 mg of prednisone. But the exact dosages and duration that substantially change the benefit-risk ratio for GCs varies by the personal and the underlying risk factors. The risk factors for infections are the underlying disorders (especially rheumatoid arthritis and systemic lupus erythematosus), patient age, lower functional status, and concomitant use of immunosuppressive or biologic therapies. In addition, a low albumin level is strongly associated with the risk of infection, because of direct (i.e. as an etiological factor) or indirect (i.e. by being a marker of the malnutrition-inflammation syndrome) effects. Furthermore, a low albumin level is associated with a higher free glucocorticoid fraction. Due to the inhibition of cytokine release and associated reduction in inflammatory and febrile responses, patients treated with GCs may not be presented with obvious signs and symptoms of infection. Therefore, it may be difficult to detect infections at an early stage. In addition to serious bacterial infections, the increase in risk is much higher for opportunistic infections (e.g. *Pneumocystis jiroveci* pneumonia, herpes zoster tuberculosis, listeriosis, aspergillosis, nontuberculous mycobacterial disease, invasive fungal infections), and in specific populations (e.g. allogeneic bone marrow transplant and solid organ transplant). Reactivation of cytomegalovirus with GCs is a serious problem especially in solid organ transplant recipients [127–131].

Lymphocytes	**Monocytes/macrophages**
• Reversible lymphopenia, CD4 depletion (>50% reduction) • Decreased proliferation and migration of lymphocytes • Impaired delayed-type hypersensitivity • Impaired natural killer cell cytotoxicity • Decreased lymphokine production (interleukin-2, TNFα,interleukin-12, interferon γ) • Th1/Th2 dysregulation of T-helper cells (decreased Th1 and increased Th2 cytokine production) • Impaired phagocyte effector cell function and cellular immune response	• Reversible monocytopenia (>40% reduction) • Impaired phagocytosis and oxidative killing • Decreased chemotaxis and migration to sites of inflammation • Impaired formation of nitric oxide • Impaired maturation of monocytes to macrophages • Inhibition of pro-inflammatory cytokine production(interleukin-1, interleukin-6, TNFα)
Neutrophils	**Other immune effector cells**
• Impaired phagocytosis, degranulation, and oxidative burst • Reduced cytokine production • Impaired formation of nitric oxide • Defective adherence to endothelium, extravasation,chemotaxis • Inhibition of apoptosis	• Decreased counts for alveolar dendritic cells, central nervous system microglial cells, and Langerhans' epidermal cells • Impaired antigen-presenting capacity of dendritic and Langerhans' cells (decreased expression of MHC II on their surface) • Defective microglial cell-killing capacity (impaired nitric oxide formation)
Other effects	
• Inhibition of prostaglandin production • Inhibition of host's inflammatory response • Attenuation of clinical (i.e. fever) and radiological signs of infection • Potential delay of diagnosis	

Table 9. Immunosuppressive effects of glucocorticoids (adapted from [126]).

15. Myopathy

GCs have direct catabolic effects on skeletal muscles. These catabolic effects are mediated by several cellular mechanisms. GCs inhibit the glucose uptake in skeletal muscles, by this way stimulate protein catabolism and inhibit protein synthesis in muscles. These direct effects causes muscle weakness. Besides, it was shown that GCs increase the transcription of genes encoding components of the ubiquitin-proteasome pathway, thereby increasing the proteolytic capacity of muscle cells. Transactivation of certain genes through glucocorticoid receptors also contributes to muscle atrophy. GCs inhibit the production by the muscle of IGF-I, a growth factor that stimulates the development of muscle mass by increasing protein synthesis and myogenesis, while decreasing proteolysis and apoptosis. In addition, GCs stimulate the production of myostatin, a growth factor that inhibits the muscle mass development by downregulating the proliferation and protein synthesis [132–135].

Myopathy usually develops over several weeks to months with the use of GCs. The typical clinical features are proximal muscle weakness and atrophy in both the upper and lower extremities. Quadriceps and other pelvic girdle muscles are more severely affected. Myalgias and muscle tenderness are not seen. Although there is some variation in the dose and duration of GCs prior to the onset of muscle weakness, the higher the dose of GCs used related with the more rapid the onset. But it is more common in patients treated with ≥10 mg/day of prednisone or equivalent. The severity and the mechanism for the catabolic effect of GCs may differ with age. Creatine phosphokinase, aldolase, aspartate aminotransferase, lactate dehydrogenase (LDH), LDH isoenzymes, and changes in urinary excretion of creatine neither correlate with the degree of muscle weakness, nor discriminate between patients receiving small and large doses of GCs. So there is no definitive diagnostic test for myopathy induced by GCs. Diagnosis is to exclude other possible etiologic factors. Weakness of peripheral and respiratory muscles may have significant clinical effects, such as loss of quality of life, fatigue, impaired wound healing, compromised lung function, and poor immune response. Treatment is discontinuation of GCs or dose reductions immediately. Symptoms generally improve within 3–4 weeks of dose reductions, and often resolve after discontinuation of GCs [136–138].

16. Cutaneous side effects

The most important cutaneous side effects of systemic GCs are skin atrophy-fragility, irreversible striae rubrae distensae (red striae), purpura, and delayed wound healing. A rare but unimportant side effect is hypertrichosis. Fortunately, hypertrichosis is usually reversible and disappears after discontinuation of GCs. The potency and duration of therapy determine the occurrence and severity of cutaneous lesions.

16.1. Skin atrophy

All parts of the skin involved become thin and fragile. Women seem to be more susceptible to this side effect. Suppression of cutaneous cell proliferation and protein synthesis causes skin atrophy. Further effects of GCs on the skin are a decreased synthesis of epidermal lipids, as well as an increased transepidermal water loss [139, 140].

16.2. Striae

These are visible linear scars that form in areas of dermal damage, presumably during mechanical stress. Stria means scar tissue. For this reason, once developed, they are permanent. In the differential diagnosis, excessive weight gain and pregnancy should be excluded [141].

16.3. Delayed wound healing

The effects of GCs on wound healing are multifactorial. GCs prevent the early inflammatory phase, which is essential for wound repair. GCs also affect keratinocytes (epidermal atrophy and delayed reepithelialization), fibroblasts (reduced collagen and ground substance, resulting in dermal atrophy, and striae), and vascular connective tissue support (telangiectasia, purpura, and easy bruising). According to delayed granulation, tissue formation of GCs impairs angiogenesis. Furthermore GCs have impact on wound healing by the regulation of pro-inflammatory cytokines, growth factors, matrix proteins, and matrix proteases [142].

16.4. Purpura

When severe dermal atrophy and loss of intercellular substance occur by GCs, blood vessels lose their surrounding dermal matrix. The fragility of dermal vessels causes purpura. The dorsum of the hands, forearms, sides of the neck, face, and lower legs (sun exposed areas) are the most common affected sites [143].

17. Psychiatric and cognitive disturbances

Systemic GCs induce dose-dependent a wide range of psychiatric and cognitive disturbances, including memory impairment, agitation, anxiety, fear, hypomania, insomnia, irritability, lethargy, mood lability, and even psychosis [144].

17.1. Behavioral effects

Increase in appetite resulting with weight gain is the most common behavioral side effect of long-term exposure to GCs. Weight gain does not correlate with the cumulative dose. Sleep disturbances are the second most common behavioral side effects of GCs and dose-dependent. The evening dose induces sleeplessness [145, 146].

17.2. Psychic effects

Psychic side effects (PSE) of GCs are quantitatively/qualitatively distinct forms. Symptoms range from an initial slight increase in the overall sense of well-being (independent of improvement in their underlying disease activity) or low-grade mood changes, such as euphoria, grandiosity, emotional lability, depressed or elated mood, up to severe psychiatric disorders, and suicidality. The frequency ranges from 1.3 to 62% in adults. The predicted threshold dose for PSE is ≥20 mg/day of prednisone (or equivalent), but can be seen at very low dosages. PSE commonly develop within the first weeks of exposure, but may occur within few days or at any point during treatment, including withdrawal (especially after long-term and high dose exposures). A family history of depression, previous neuropsychiatric disorders, and alcoholism has also been reported as risk factors for the development of PSE. Women were more likely to develop depression, whereas men were more likely to develop mania. The risk of depression, mania, delirium, confusion, and disorientation increases, but suicidal behavior and panic disorder decreases with age. PSE often disappears shortly after dose reduction or discontinuation. Switching to alternative GCs may be helpful. Clinicians should ask about a prior history of psychiatric disorder and refer patients to a psychiatrist [147–149].

17.3. Cognitive effects

Cognitive impairment is a common, dose-dependent side effect of GCs. Common symptoms are deficits in attention, concentration, memory retention, mental speed, and efficiency. Prolonged exposure to moderate/high doses of GCs may cause cumulative and long-lasting effects on specific brain areas. Low doses of GCs do not affect adult cognitive functions in both short- and long-term exposure. Older patients appear to be more sensitive to memory impairment with short-term exposure [149].

http://dx.doi.org/10.5772/intechopen.72019

18. Monitoring and prevention of side effects

The same total dose of GCs among systemic treatments has different side effects. Split-dose regimens are more toxic than single daily-dose protocols. Both these protocols are more toxic than alternate-day treatment programs. In daily treatment regimens, SGCs with long biologic half-lives (e.g. dexamethasone) have a greater potential for side effects than analogs do with intermediate biologic half-lives (e.g. prednisone). High doses of systemic GCs can be administered for less than a week with partial safety, even though the same dose of drug administered for a more prolonged period will result in presumably, clinically significant side effects. The lowest dose of GCs should be used for the shortest period of time that is needed to achieve the treatment goals. Preexisting comorbid conditions (diabetes mellitus, hypertension, dyslipidemia, heart failure, cataract or glaucoma, peptic ulcer disease, use of nonsteroidal anti-inflammatory drugs, low bone density, or osteoporosis) may increase risk when GCs are required. To provide an optimal therapy, patient education is very important. Patients should be informed about the side effects of GCs. GCs generally stimulate the appetite, causes weight gain, elevated blood pressure, and glucose levels. Therefore, patients should be informed about the importance of diet when therapy is begun. The symptoms and signs of side effects related with GCs, should also be explained to the patients [32, 51–53]. For systemic therapy, the choice of specific GCs depends, partially, on clinical variables like underlying or accompanying diseases. Hydrocortisone is usually used for physiologic replacement and "stress" coverage in patients with HPA suppression. Hydrocortisone has a short biologic half-life and causes sodium and potassium retention. Thus, this agent is not commonly used for systemic immunosuppressive or anti-inflammatory treatment. Fluorinated analogs, such as dexamethasone, have a long biologic half-life and little sodium-retaining potency. But long biologic half-life, may be associated with a greater potential for side effects. As a result, this group of SGCs is not commonly used in prolonged daily therapy regimens [54].

19. Concluding remarks

To reduce the incidence and severity of these side effects (described above); they should be well known. Besides, dose of GCs should be decreased carefully. According to the patients' risk factors taking general preventive measures are important.

Author details

Irmak Sayın Alan[1*] and Bahadır Alan[2]

*Address all correspondence to: irmaksayin@yahoo.com

1 Okan University, Medical Faculty, Department of Internal Medicine, Istanbul, Turkey

2 Okan University, Medical Faculty, Department of Cardiology, Istanbul, Turkey

References

[1] Liu D, Ahmet A, Ward L, Krishnamoorthy P, Mandelcorn ED, Leigh R, Brown JP, Cohen A, Kim H. A practical guide to the monitoring and management of the complications of systemic corticosteroid therapy. Allergy, Asthma and Clinical Immunology. 2013 Aug 15;**9**(1):30. DOI: 10.1186/1710-1492-9-30

[2] Pousseau GG, Baxter JD, Tomkins GP. Glucocorticoid receptor: Relation between steroid binding and biologic effects. Journal of Molecular Biology. 1972;**67**:99-115

[3] Magiakou MA, Chrousos GP. Corticosteroid therapy, nonendocrine disease and corticosteroid withdrawal. In: Bardin CW, editor. Current Therapy in Endocrinology and Metabolism. 5th ed. Philadelphia: Mosby Yearbook; 1994. pp. 120-124

[4] Magiakou MA, Chrousos GP. Corticosteroid therapy and withdrawal. In: Endocrinology and Metabolic Diseases, Current Practice of Medicine. Philadelphia; 1996. pp. IV: 6.1-6.6

[5] Liapi C, Chrousos GP. Glucocorticoids. In: Jaffe SJ, Aranda JV, editors. Pediatric Pharmacology. 2nd ed. Philadelphia: WB Saunders Co; 1992. pp. 466-475

[6] Chrousos GP. Adrenocorticosteroids & adrenocortical antagonists. In: Katzung BG, editor. Basic & Clinical Pharmacology. 10th ed. New York, NY: McGraw-Hill Medical; 2007. pp. 635-652

[7] Stewart PM. The adrenal cortex. In: Kronenberg HM, Melmed S, Polonsky KS, Larsen RP, editors. Williams Textbook of Endocrinology. 11th ed. Philadelphia, PA: Saunders; 2008: Chapter 14

[8] Migeon CJ, Lawrence B, Bertrand J, Holman GH. In vivo distribution of some 17-hydroxycorticoids between the plasma and red blood cells of man. The Journal of Clinical Endocrinology and Metabolism. 1959;**19**:1411

[9] Pugeat MM, Dunn JF, Nisula BC. Transport of steroid hormones: Interaction of 70 drugs with testosterone-binding globulin and corticosteroid-binding globulin in human plasma. The Journal of Clinical Endocrinology and Metabolism. 1981;**53**:69

[10] Ballard PL. Delivery and transport of glucocorticoids to target cells. In: Rousseau GG (Eds), Glucocorticoid Hormone Action, Baxter JD, Springer-Verlag, Berlin 1979. p. 25

[11] Peterson RE. Metabolism of adrenocorticosteroids in man. Annals of the New York Academy of Sciences. 1959;**82**:846

[12] Goodwin JS. Antiinflammatory drugs. In: Stites DP, Terr AI, Parslow TG, editors. Basic and Clinical Immunology. 8th ed. East Norwalk: Appleton and Lange; 1994. pp. 786-795

[13] Winkelstein A. Immunosuppressive therapy. In: Stites DP, Terr AT, Parslow TG, editors. Basic and Clinical Immunology. 8th ed. San Mateo: Appleton and Lange; 1994. pp. 767-780

[14] Schacke H, Docke WD, Asadullah K. Mechanisms involved in the side effects of glucocorticoids. Pharmacology & Therapeutics. 2002 Oct;**96**(1):23-43

[15] Frampton AE, Eynon CA. High dose methylprednisolone in the immediate management of acute, blunt spinal cord injury: What is the current practice in emergency departments, spinal units, and neurosurgical units in the UK? Emergency Medicine Journal. 2006 Jul;**23**(7):550-553

[16] Salerno A, Hermann R. Efficacy and safety of steroid use for postoperative pain relief. Update and review of the medical literature. The Journal of Bone and Joint Surgery. American Volume. 2006 Jun;**88**(6):1361-1372

[17] Tegethoff M, Pryce C, Meinlschmidt G. Effects of intrauterine exposure to synthetic glucocorticoids on fetal, newborn, and infant hypothalamic-pituitary-adrenal axis function in humans: A systematic review. Endocrine Reviews. 2009 Dec;**30**(7):753-789

[18] Gross AK, Winstead PS. Current controversies in critical illness-related corticosteroid insufficiency and glucocorticoid supplementation. Orthopedics. 2009 Sep;**32**(9)

[19] Liu D, Ahmet A, Ward L, Krishnamoorthy P, Mandelcorn ED, Leigh R, Brown JP, Cohen A, Kim HA. Practical guide to the monitoring and management of the complications of systemic corticosteroid therapy. Allergy, Asthma and Clinical Immunology. 2013 Aug 15;**9**(1):30

[20] Boumpas DT, Chrousos GP, Wilder RL, Cupps TR, Balow JE. Glucocorticoid therapy for immune-mediated diseases: Basic and clinical correlates. Annals of Internal Medicine. 1993 Dec 15;**119**(12):1198-1208

[21] Scheinman RI, Cogswell PC, Lofquist AK, Baldwin AS Jr. Role of transcriptional activation of I kappa B alpha in mediation of immunosuppression by glucocorticoids. Science 1995;**270**:283

[22] Auphan N, DiDonato JA, Rosette C, et al. Immunosuppression by glucocorticoids: Inhibition of NF-kappa B activity through induction of I kappa B synthesis. Science. 1995;**270**:286

[23] Rhen T, Cidlowski JA. Antiinflammatory action of glucocorticoids--new mechanisms for old drugs. The New England Journal of Medicine. 2005;**353**:1711

[24] Fan PT, DT Y, Clements PJ, et al. Effect of corticosteroids on the human immune response: Comparison of one and three daily 1 gm intravenous pulses of methylprednisolone. The Journal of Laboratory and Clinical Medicine. 1978;**91**:625

[25] Fauci AS, Dale DC, Balow JE. Glucocorticosteroid therapy: Mechanisms of action and clinical considerations. Annals of Internal Medicine. 1976;**84**:304

[26] Sternberg EM, Wilder RL. Corticosteroids. In: McCarty DJ, Koopman WJ, editors. Arthritis and Allied Conditions. Philadelphia: Lea & Febiger; 1993. pp. 665-682

[27] Sternberg EM, Chrousos GP, Wilder RL, Gold PW. The stress response and the regulation of inflammatory disease. Annals of Internal Medicine. 1992;**117**:854-866

[28] Sternberg EM, Wilder RL. Corticosteroids. In: McCarty DJ, Koopman WJ, editors. Arthritis and Allied Conditions. Philadelphia: Lea & Febiger; 1993. pp. 665-682

[29] Wang J, Wang R, Wang H, Yang X, Yang J, Xiong W, Wen Q, Ma L. Glucocorticoids suppress antimicrobial autophagy and nitric oxide production and facilitate mycobacterial survival in macrophages. Scientific Reports. 2017 Apr 20;**7**(1):982

[30] van de Garde MD, Martinez FO, Melgert BN, Hylkema MN, Jonkers RE, Hamann J. Chronic exposure to glucocorticoids shapes gene expression and modulates innate and adaptive activation pathways in macrophages with distinct changes in leukocyte attraction. Journal of Immunology. 2014 Feb 1;**192**(3):1196-1208

[31] Rinehart JJ, Sagone AL, Balcerzak SP, et al. Effects of corticosteroid therapy on human monocyte function. The New England Journal of Medicine. 1975;**292**:236

[32] Wallen N, Kita H, Weiler D, Gleich GJ. Glucocorticoids inhibit cytokine-mediated eosinophil survival. Journal of Immunology. 1991;**147**:3490

[33] Park SK, Beaven MA. Mechanism of upregulation of the inhibitory regulator, src-like adaptor protein (SLAP), by glucocorticoids in mast cells. Molecular Immunology. 2009; **46**:492

[34] Eddy JL, Krukowski K, Janusek L, Mathews HL. Glucocorticoids regulate natural killer cell function epigenetically. Cellular Immunology. 2014;**290**:120

[35] Fauci AS, Dale DC. The effect of in vivo hydrocortisone on subpopulations of human lymphocytes. The Journal of Clinical Investigation. 1974 Jan;**53**(1):240-246

[36] Paliogianni F, Ahuja SS, Balow JP, Balow JE, Boumpas DT. Novel mechanism for inhibition of T cells by glucocorticoids (GC): GC modulate signal transduction through IL-2 receptor. Journal of Immunology. 1993;**151**:4081-4089

[37] Franchimont D, Louis E, Dewe W, et al. Effects of dexamethasone on the profile of cytokine secretion in human whole blood cell cultures. Regulatory Peptides. 1998;**73**:59

[38] Ashwell JD, FW L, Vacchio MS. Glucocorticoids in T cell development and function*. Annual Review of Immunology. 2000;**18**:309

[39] Cupps TR, Gerrard TL, Falkoff RJ, Whalen G, Fauci AS. Effects of in vitro corticosteroids on B cell activation, proliferation, and differentiation. The Journal of Clinical Investigation. 1985 Feb;**75**(2):754-761

[40] Butler WT, Rossen RD. Effects of corticosteroids on immunity in man: Decreased serum IgG concentration caused by 3 or 5 days of high doses of methylprednisolone. The Journal of Clinical Investigation. 1973;**52**:2629-2640

[41] Shiao RT, McLeskey SB, Khera SY, Wolfson A, Freter CE. Mechanisms of inhibition of IL-6-mediated immunoglobulin secretion by dexamethasone and suramin in human lymphoid and myeloma cell lines. Leukemia & Lymphoma. 1996 Apr;**21**(3-4):293-303

[42] Levy AL, Waldmann TA. The effect of hydrocortisone on immunoglobulin metabolism. The Journal of Clinical Investigation. 1970;**49**:1679

[43] Jabara HH, Ahern DJ, Vercelli D, Geha RS. Hydrocortisone and IL-4 induce IgE isotype switching in human B cells. Journal of Immunology. 1991;**147**:1557

[44] Shodell M, Shah K, Siegal FP. Circulating human plasmacytoid dendritic cells are highly sensitive to corticosteroid administration. Lupus. 2003;**12**:222

[45] Gadson PF, Russell JD, Russell SB. Glucocorticoid receptors in human fibroblasts derived from normal dermis and keloid tissue. The Journal of Biological Chemistry. 1984;**259**: 11236-11241

[46] Meisler N et al. Dexamethasone abrogates the fibrogenic effect of transforming growth factor-beta in rat granuloma and granulation tissue fibroblasts. The Journal of Investigative Dermatology. 1997;**108**:285-289

[47] Bailey JM. New mechanisms for effects of anti-inflammatory glucocorticoids. BioFactors. 1991;**3**:97-102

[48] Mukherjee AB, Cordella-Miele E, Miele L. Regulation of extracellular phospholipase A2 activity: Implications for inflammatory diseases. DNA and Cell Biology. 1992;**11**:233-243

[49] Masferrer JL, Seibert K, Zweifel B, Needleman P. Endogenous glucocorticoids regulate an inducible cyclooxygenase enzyme. Proceedings of the National Academy of Sciences of the United States of America. 1992;**89**:3917-3921

[50] O'Banion MK, Winn VD, Young DA. cDNA cloning and functional activity of a glucocorticoid-regulated inflammatory cyclooxygenase. Proceedings of the National Academy of Sciences of the United States of America. 1992;**89**:4888-4892

[51] D'Adamio F, Zollo O, Moraca R, Ayroldi E, Bruscoli S, Bartoli A, et al. A new dexamethasone-induced gene of the leucine zipper family protects T lymphocytes from TCR/CD3-activated cell death. Immunity. 1997;**7**:803-812

[52] Lim W, Park C, Shim MK, Lee YH, Lee YM, Lee Y. Glucocorticoids suppress hypoxia-induced COX-2 and hypoxia inducible factor-1α expression through the induction of glucocorticoid-induced leucine zipper. British Journal of Pharmacology. 2014 Feb; **171**(3):735-745

[53] Yang N, Zhang W, Shi XM. Glucocorticoid-induced leucine zipper (GILZ) mediates glucocorticoid action and inhibits inflammatory cytokine-induced COX-2 expression. Journal of Cellular Biochemistry. 2008;**103**:1760-1771

[54] Huscher D, Thiele K, Gromnica-Ihle E, Hein G, Demary W, Dreher R, Zink A, Buttgereit F. Dose-related patterns of glucocorticoid-induced side effects. Annals of the Rheumatic Diseases. 2009 Jul;**68**(7):1119-1124

[55] Da Silva JA, Jacobs JW, Kirwan JR, Boers M, Saag KG, Inês LB, de Koning EJ, Buttgereit F, Cutolo M, Capell H, Rau R, Bijlsma JW. Safety of low dose glucocorticoid treatment in rheumatoid arthritis: Published evidence and prospective trial data. Annals of the Rheumatic Diseases. 2006 Mar;**65**(3):285-293

[56] McDonough AK, Curtis JR, Saag KG. The epidemiology of glucocorticoid-associated adverse events. Current Opinion in Rheumatology. 2008 Mar;**20**(2):131-137

[57] Krasner AS. Glucocorticoid-induced adrenal insufficiency. Journal of the American Medical Association. 1999 Aug 18;**282**(7):671-676

[58] Sorkness CA, LaForce C, Storms W, Lincourt WR, Edwards L, Rogenes PR. Effects of the inhaled corticosteroids fluticasone propionate, triamcinolone acetonide, and flunisolide and oral prednisone on the hypothalamic-pituitary-adrenal axis in adult patients with asthma. Clinical Therapeutics. 1999;**21**(2):353-367

[59] Schimmer BP, Funder JW. ACTH. Adrenal steroids and pharmacology of the adrenal cortex. In: Brunton LL, Chabner BA, Knollmann BC, editors. Goodman and Gilman's the Pharmacological Basis of Therapeutics. 12th ed. New York, NY: McGraw-Hill Companies Inc; 2011

[60] Stewart PM, Krone NP. The adrenal cortex. In: Melmed S, Polonsky KS, Larsen PR, Kronenberg HM, editors. Williams Textbook of Endocrinology. 12th ed. Philadelphia, Pa: Saunders Elsevier; 2011

[61] Park SH, Cho KH. Large-dose glucocorticoid induced secondary adrenal insufficiency in spinal cord injury. Annals of Rehabilitation Medicine. 2016 Dec;**40**(6):1033-1039

[62] Ortega E, Rodriguez C, Strand LJ, Segre E. Effects of cloprednol and other corticosteroids on hypothalamic-pituitary-adrenal axis function. The Journal of International Medical Research. 1976;**4**:326-337

[63] Axelrod L. Corticosteroid therapy. In: Becker KL, editor. Principles and Practice of Endocrinology and Metabolism. 3rd ed. Philadelphia, PA: Lippincott Williams and Wilkins; 2000. pp. 752-763

[64] Buttgereit F, da Silva JA, Boers M, Burmester GR, Cutolo M, Jacobs J, Kirwan J, Kohler L, Van Riel P, Vischer T, Bijlsma JW: Standardised nomenclature for glucocorticoid dosages and glucocorticoid treatment regimens: Current questions and tentative answers in rheumatology. Annals of the Rheumatic Diseases 2002;**61**:718-722

[65] Axelrod L. Glucocorticoid therapy. Medicine (Baltimore). 1976 Jan;**55**(1):39-65

[66] Schürmeyer TH, Tsokos GC, Avgerinos PC, et al. Pituitary-adrenal responsiveness to corticotropin-releasing hormone in patients receiving chronic, alternate day glucocorticoid therapy. The Journal of Clinical Endocrinology and Metabolism. 1985;**61**:22-27

[67] Bell NH. The glucocorticoid withdrawal syndrome. Advances in Experimental Medicine and Biology. 1984;**171**:293-299

[68] Glowniak JV, Loriaux DL. A double-blind study of perioperative steroid requirements in secondary adrenal insufficiency. Surgery. 1997;**121**:123-129

[69] Fardet L, Fève B. Systemic glucocorticoid therapy: A review of its metabolic and cardiovascular adverse events. Drugs. 2014 Oct;**74**(15):1731-1745

[70] Curtis JR, Westfall AO, Allison J, et al. Population-based assessment of adverse events associated with long-term glucocorticoid use. Arthritis and Rheumatism. 2006; **55**(3):420-426

[71] Fardet L, Cabane J, Lebbe C, Morel P, Flahault A. Incidence and risk factors for corticosteroid-induced lipodystrophy: A prospective study. Journal of the American Academy of Dermatology. 2007;**57**(4):604-609

[72] Horber FF, Zürcher RM, Herren H, Crivelli MA, Robotti G, Frey FJ. Altered body fat distribution in patients with glucocorticoid treatment and in patients on long-term dialysis. The American Journal of Clinical Nutrition. 1986;**43**(5):758-769

[73] Huscher D, Thiele K, Gromnica-Ihle E, et al. Dose-related patterns of glucocorticoid-induced side effects. Annals of the Rheumatic Diseases. 2009;**68**(7):1119-1124

[74] Fardet L, Antuna-Puente B, Vatier C, et al. Adipokine profile in glucocorticoid-treated patients: Baseline plasma leptin level predicts occurrence of lipodystrophy. Clinical Endocrinology. 2013;**78**(1):43-51

[75] Wei L, MacDonald TM, Walker BR. Taking glucocorticoids by prescription is associated with subsequent cardiovascular disease. Annals of Internal Medicine. 2004; **141**(10):764-770

[76] Souverein PC, Berard A, Van Staa TP, et al. Use of oral glucocorticoids and risk of cardiovascular and cerebrovascular disease in a population based case-control study. Heart. 2004;**90**(8):859-865

[77] Davis JM, Kremers HM, Crowson CS, Nicola PJ, Ballman KV, Therneau TM, et al. Glucocorticoids and cardiovascular events in rheumatoid arthritis – A population-based cohort study. Arthritis and Rheumatism. 2007;**56**:820-830

[78] Christiansen CF, Christensen S, Mehnert F, Cummings SR, Chapurlat RD, Sørensen HT. Glucocorticoid use and risk of atrial fibrillation or flutter: A population-based, case-control study. Archives of Internal Medicine. 2009 Oct 12;**169**(18):1677-1683

[79] Ren R, Oakley RH, Cruz-Topete D, Cidlowski JA. Dual role for glucocorticoids in cardiomyocyte hypertrophy and apoptosis. Endocrinology. 2012;**153**(11):5346-5360

[80] Armstrong KA, Hiremagalur B, Haluska BA, Campbell SB, Hawley CM, Marks L, et al. Free fatty acids are associated with obesity, insulin resistance, and atherosclerosis in renal transplant recipients. Transplantation. 2005;**80**:937-944

[81] Beentjes JAM, Van Tol A, Sluiter WJ, Dullaart RPF. Decreased plasma cholesterol esterification and cholesteryl ester transfer in hypopituitary patients on glucocorticoid replacement therapy. Scandinavian Journal of Clinical and Laboratory Investigation. 2000;**60**:189-198

[82] del Rincon I, O'Leary DH, Haas RW, Escalante A. Effect of glucocorticoids on the arteries in rheumatoid arthritis. Arthritis and Rheumatism. 2004;**50**:3813-3822

[83] Costenbader KH, Liang MH, Chibnik LB, Aizer J, Kwon H, Gall V, et al. A pravastatin dose-escalation study in systemic lupus erythematosus. Rheumatology International. 2007;**27**:1071-1077

[84] Burt MG, Roberts GW, Aguilar-Loza NR, Frith P, Stranks SN. Continuous monitoring of circadian glycemic patterns in patients receiving prednisolone for COPD. The Journal of Clinical Endocrinology and Metabolism. 2011;**96**:1789-1796

[85] Donihi AC, Raval D, Saul M, Korytkowski MT, DeVita MA. Prevalence and predictors of corticosteroid-related hyperglycemia in hospitalized patients. Endocrine Practice. 2006;**12**:358-362

[86] Gulliford MC, Charlton J, Latinovic R. Risk of diabetes associated with prescribed glucocorticoids in a large population. Diabetes Care. 2006;**29**(12):2728-2729

[87] Feldman-Billard S, Lissak B, Kassaei R, Benrabah R, Héron E. Short-term tolerance of pulse methylprednisolone therapy in patients with diabetes mellitus. Ophthalmology. 2005;**112**(3):511-515

[88] Schneiter P, Tappy L. Kinetics of dexamethasone-induced alterations of glucose metabolism in healthy humans. The American Journal of Physiology. 1998;**275**:E806-E813

[89] Gurwitz JH, Bohn RL, Glynn RJ, Monane M, Mogun H, Avorn J. Glucocorticoids and the risk for initiation of hypoglycemic therapy. Archives of Internal Medicine. 1994;**154**:97-101

[90] Spinola-Castro AM, Siviero-Miachon AA, Andreoni S, Tosta-Hernandez PD, Macedo CR, Lee ML. Transient hyperglycemia during childhood acute lymphocytic leukemia chemotherapy: An old event revisited. Clinical Advances in Hematology & Oncology. 2009;**7**:465-472

[91] Clore JN, Thurby-Hay L. Glucocorticoid-induced hyperglycemia. Endocrine Practice. 2009;**15**:469-474

[92] Weinstein SP, Wilson CM, Pritsker A, Cushman SW. Dexamethasone inhibits insulin-stimulated recruitment of GLUT4 to the cell surface in rat skeletal muscle. Metabolism. 1998;**47**:3-6

[93] van Raalte DH, Ouwens DM, Diamant M. Novel insights into glucocorticoid-mediated diabetogenic effects: Towards expansion of therapeutic options? European Journal of Clinical Investigation. 2009;**39**:81-93

[94] Cadoudal T, Leroyer S, Reis AF, et al. Proposed involvement of adipocyte glyceroneogenesis and phosphoenolpyruvate carboxykinase in the metabolic syndrome. Biochimie. 2005;**87**:27-32

[95] Beaudry JL, Riddell MC. Effects of glucocorticoids and exercise on pancreatic b-cell function and diabetes development. Diabetes/Metabolism Research and Reviews. 2012; **28**(7):560-573

[96] Gremlich S, Roduit R, Thorens B. Dexamethasone induces posttranslational degradation of GLUT2 and inhibition of insülin secretion in isolated pancreatic beta cells. Comparison with the effects of fatty acids. The Journal of Biological Chemistry. 1997; **272**(6):3216-3222

[97] Hansen KB, Vilsbøll T, Bagger JI, Holst JJ, Knop FK. Reduced glucose tolerance and insulin resistance induced by steroid treatment, relative physical inactivity, and high-calorie diet impairs the incretin effect in healthy subjects. The Journal of Clinical Endocrinology and Metabolism. 2010;**95**(7):3309-3317

[98] Kanis JA, Johansson H, Oden A, Johnell O, de Laet C, Melton LJ III, Tenenhouse A, Reeve J, Silman AJ, Pols HA, Eisman JA, McCloskey EV, Mellstrom D. A meta-analysis of prior corticosteroid use and fracture risk. Journal of Bone and Mineral Research. 2004;**19**:893-899

[99] Robert S, Weinstein MD. Glucocorticoid-induced osteoporosis and osteonecrosis. Endocrinology and Metabolism Clinics of North America. 2012 September;**41**(3): 595-611

[100] Reid IR. Glucocorticoid-induced osteoporosis. Baillière's Clinical Endocrinology and Metabolism. 2000;**14**:279-298

[101] Weinstein RS, Jilka RL, Parfitt AM, Manolagas SC. Inhibition of osteoblastogenesis and promotion of apoptosis of osteoblasts and osteocytes by glucocorticoids. Potential mechanisms of their deleterious effects on bone. The Journal of Clinical Investigation. 1998;**102**:274-282

[102] Yao W, Cheng Z, Busse C, Pham A, Nakamura MC, Lane NE. Glucocorticoid excess in mice results in early activation of osteoclastogenesis and adipogenesis and prolonged suppression of osteogenesis: A longitudinal study of gene expression in bone tissue from glucocorticoid-treated mice. Arthritis and Rheumatism. 2008;**58**:1674-1686

[103] Canalis E, Delany AM. Mechanisms of glucocorticoid action in bone. Annals of the New York Academy of Sciences. 2002;**966**:73-81

[104] Weinstein RS. Glucocorticoid-induced osteonecrosis. Endocrine. 2012 Apr;**41**(2):183-190

[105] Kaste SC, Karimova EJ, Neel MD. Osteonecrosis in children after therapy for malignancy. American Journal of Roentgenology. 2011;**196**:1011-1018

[106] Barr RD, Sala A. Osteonecrosis in children and adolescents with cancer. Pediatric Blood & Cancer. 2008;**50**(2 Suppl):483-485

[107] WHO. World Health Organization (WHO): Fact sheet #317: Cardiovascular diseases (CVDs); 2013

[108] Ferrari P, Krozowski Z. Role of the 11b-hydroxysteroid dehydrogenase type 2 in blood pressure regulation. Kidney International. 2000;**57**:1374-1381

[109] Baum M, Moe OW. Glucocorticoid-mediated hypertension: Does the vascular smooth muscle hold all the answers? Journal of the American Society of Nephrology. 2008;**19**:1251-1253

[110] Sato A, Funder JW, Okubo M, Kubota E, Saruta T. Glucocorticoid-induced hypertension in the elderly. Relation to serum calcium and family history of essential hypertension. American Journal of Hypertension. 1995;**8**(8):823-828

[111] Choi HK, Seeger JD. Glucocorticoid use and serum lipid levels in US adults: The third National Health and nutrition examination survey. Arthritis and Rheumatism. 2005;**53**(4):528-535

[112] Zimmerman J, Fainaru M, Eisenberg S. The effects of prednisone therapy on plasma lipoproteins and apolipoproteins: A prospective study. Metabolism, Clinical and Experimental. 1984;**33**(6):521-526

[113] Ettinger WH, Klinefelter HF, Kwiterovitch PO. Effect of shortterm, low-dose corticosteroids on plasma lipoprotein lipids. Atherosclerosis. 1987;**63**(2-3):167-172

[114] Svenson KL, Lithell H, Hällgren R, Vessby B. Serum lipoprotein in active rheumatoid arthritis and other chronic inflammatory arthritides. II. Effects of anti-inflammatory and disease-modifying drug treatment. Archives of Internal Medicine. 1987;**147**:1917-1920

[115] Arnaldi G, Scandali VM, Trementino L, Cardinaletti M, Appolloni G, Boscaro M. Pathophysiology of Dyslipidemia in Cushing's syndrome. Neuroendocrinology. 2010;**92**(suppl 1):86-90

[116] Piper JM, Ray WA, Daugherty JR, Griffin MR. Corticosteroid use and peptic ulcer disease: Role of nonsteroidal anti-inflammatory drugs. Annals of Internal Medicine. 1991;**114**:735-740

[117] Conn HO, Poynard T. Corticosteroids and peptic ulcer: Meta-analysis of adverse events during steroid therapy. Journal of Internal Medicine. 1994;**236**:619-632

[118] Richardson CT. Pathogenetic factors in peptic ulcer disease. The American Journal of Medicine. 1985;**79**:1-7

[119] Narum S, Westergren T, Klemp M. Corticosteroids and risk of gastrointestinal bleeding: A systematic review and meta-analysis. BMJ Open. 2014;**4**:e004587

[120] Hernández-Díaz S, Rodríguez LA. Steroids and risk of upper gastrointestinal complications. American Journal of Epidemiology. 2001;**153**:1089-1093

[121] Sadr-Azodi O, Mattsson F, Bexlius TS, Lindblad M, Lagergren J, Ljung R. Association of oral glucocorticoid use with an increased risk of acute pancreatitis: A population-based nested case-control study. JAMA Internal Medicine. 2013 Mar 25;**173**(6):444-449

[122] Garbe E, Lelorier J, Boivin JF, Suissa S. Risk of ocular hypertension or open-angle glaucoma in elderly patients on oral glucocorticoids. Lancet. 1997;**350**:979-982

[123] Tripathi RC, Parapuram SK, Tripathi BJ, Zhong Y, Chalam KV. Corticosteroids and glaucoma risk. Drugs & Aging. 1999;**15**:439-450

[124] Black RL, Oglesby RB, von Sallmann L, Bunim JJ. Posterior subcapsular cataracts induced by corticosteroids in patients with rheumatoid arthritis. Journal of the American Medical Association. 1960 Sep 10;**174**:166-171

[125] Haimovici R, Gragoudas ES, Duker JS, Sjaarda RN, Eliott D. Central serous chorioretinopathy associated with inhaled or intranasal corticosteroids. Ophthalmologica. 1997; **104**:1653-1660

[126] Lionakis MS, Kontoyiannis DP. Glucocorticoids and invasive fungal infections. Lancet. 2003 Nov 29;**362**(9398):1828-1838

[127] Stuck AE, Minder CE, Frey FJ. Risk of infectious complications in patients taking glucocorticosteroids. Reviews of Infectious Diseases. 1989;**11**:954-963

[128] Saag KG, Furst DE: Major side effects of systemic glucocorticoids, Up To Date 2012; 2013

[129] Saag KG. Short-term and long-term safety of glucocorticoids in rheumatoid arthritis. Bulletin of the NYU Hospital for Joint Diseases. 2012;**70**(Suppl 1):21-25

[130] Czock D, Keller F, Rasche FM, Häussler U. Pharmacokinetics and pharmacodynamics of systemically administered glucocorticoids. Clinical Pharmacokinetics. 2005;**44**:61-98

[131] Brassard P, Bitton A, Suissa A, Sinyavskaya L, Patenaude V, Suissa S. Oral corticosteroids and the risk of serious infections in patients with elderly-onset inflammatory bowel diseases. The American Journal of Gastroenterology. 2014;**109**:1795-1802

[132] LaPier TK. GC-induced muscle atrophy. The role of exercise in treatment and prevention. Journal of Cardiopulmonary Rehabilitation. 1997;**17**:76-84

[133] Price SR, Du JD, Bailey JL, Mitch WE. Molecular mechanisms regulating protein turnover in muscle. American Journal of Kidney Diseases. 2001;**37**(1 suppl. 2):S112-S114

[134] Frost RA, Lang CH. Regulation of insulin-like growth factor-I in skeletal muscle and muscle cells. Minerva Endocrinologica. 2003 Mar;**28**(1):53-73

[135] Ma K, Mallidis C, Bhasin S, Mahabadi V, Artaza J, Gonzalez-Cadavid N, Arias J, Salehian B. Glucocorticoid-induced skeletal muscle atrophy is associated with upregulation of myostatin gene expression. American Journal of Physiology Endocrinology and Metabolism. 2003 Aug;**285**(2):E363-E371

[136] Miller ML. Glucocorticoid-induced myopathy, UpToDate 2013

[137] Dardevet D, Sornet C, Savary I, Debras E, Patureau-Mirand P, Grizard J. Glucocorticoid effects on insulin- and IGF-I-regulated muscle protein metabolism during aging. The Journal of Endocrinology. 1998 Jan;**156**(1):83-89

[138] LaPier TK. Glucocorticoid-induced muscle atrophy. The role of exercise in treatment and prevention. Journal of Cardiopulmonary Rehabilitation. 1997;**17**:76-84

[139] Oikarinen A, Autio P, Kiistala U, Risteli L, Risteli J. A new method to measure type I and III collagen synthesis in human skin in vivo: Demonstration of decreased collagen synthesis after topical GC treatment. The Journal of Investigative Dermatology. 1992 Feb;**98**(2):220-225

[140] Kolbe L, Kligman AM, Schreiner V, Stoudenmayer T. Corticosteroid-induced atrophy and barrier impairment measured by non-invasive methods in human skin. Skin Research and Technology. 2001 May;**7**(2):73-77

[141] Ammar NM, Rao B, Schwartz RA, Janniger CK. Cutaneous striae. Cutis. 2000;**65**:69-70

[142] Truhan AP, Ahmed AR. Corticosteroids: A review with emphasis on complications of prolonged systemic therapy. Annals of Allergy. 1989;**62**:375-391

[143] Colomb D. Stellate spontaneous pseudoscars. Senile and presenile forms: Especially those forms caused by prolonged corticoid therapy. Archives of Dermatology. 1972;**105**:551-554

[144] Wolkowitz OM. Prospective controlled studies of the behavioral and biological effects of exogenous corticosteroids. Psychoneuroendocrinology. 1994;**19**:233-255

[145] Curtis JR, Westfall AO, Allison J, et al. Population-based assessment of adverse events associated with long-term glucocorticoid use. Arthritis and Rheumatism. 2006;**55**:420-426

[146] Wung PK, Anderson T, Fontaine KR, et al. Effects of glucocorticoids on weight change during the treatment of Wegener's granulomatosis. Arthritis and Rheumatism. 2008; **59**:746-753

[147] Fietta P, Fietta P, Delsante G. Central nervous system effects of natural and synthetic glucocorticoids. Psychiatry and Clinical Neurosciences. 2009 Oct;**63**(5):613-622

[148] Minden SL, Orav J, Schildkraut JJ. Hypomanic reactions to ACTH and prednisone treatment for multiple sclerosis. Neurology. 1988;**38**:1631-1634

[149] Fardet L, Petersen I, Nazareth I. Suicidal behavior and severe neuropsychiatric disorders following glucocorticoid therapy in primary care. The American Journal of Psychiatry. 2012;**169**:491-497

Chapter 7

New Antidepressant Medication: Benefits Versus Adverse Effects

Maria Bogdan, Eliza Gofita, Daniela Cornelia Calina, Adina Turcu-Stiolica, Anca Oana Docea, Tudor Adrian Balseanu, Adrian Camen, Gratiela Eliza Popa, Gabriela Rusu, Ina Cristofor, Liliana Pavel and Liliana Mititelu-Tartau

Additional information is available at the end of the chapter

http://dx.doi.org/10.5772/intechopen.72003

Abstract

Depression [major depressive disorder (MDD)] is a mood disturbance of multifactorial origin, associated with high rates of morbidity and mortality, lack of work productivity, adverse health behaviors, and increased healthcare expenses. MDD is a leading cause of suicide, and it affects the prognosis of chronic conditions (heart diseases, diabetes, and cancer, among others). Current pharmacological treatment for MDD covers different classes of drugs, including tricyclic antidepressants (TCAs), monoamine oxidase inhibitors (MAOIs), selective serotonin reuptake inhibitors (SSRIs), serotonin and norepinephrine reuptake inhibitors (SNRIs), and atypical antidepressants. The aim of this chapter is to review the literature, highlight the side effects of newer antidepressants, and especially point out the most important aspects of the latest agents approved for the treatment of MDD in adults: desvenlafaxine, levomilnacipran, vilazodone, and vortioxetine. Desvenlafaxine is a SNRI and the primary active metabolite of venlafaxine; also a SNRI, levomilnacipran is an enantiomer of the racemate milnacipran. Vilazodone and vortioxetine are multimodal antidepressants, which combine SSRI activity with additional receptor activity. Although they have proven efficacy in treating MDD and are being investigated for other possible indications, further detailed clinical trials are needed to establish their pharmaco-toxicological profile, following prolonged administration in patients who may suffer from various comorbidities.

Keywords: antidepressant, side effects, desvenlafaxine, levomilnacipran, vilazodone, vortioxetine

1. Introduction

Depression [major depressive disorder (MDD)] is a pathological affective disorder characterized by the presence of various emotional, physical, behavioral, and cognitive symptoms, with variable duration of manifestations, with progressive evolution toward worsening, and with a high frequency of comorbidities [1, 2].

According to the *Diagnostic and Statistical Manual of Mental Disorders*, fifth edition, the clinical symptomatology includes a series of manifestations lasting more than 2 weeks: depressed mood, diminishing interest in current activities (home and work), lack of pleasure and energy, permanent fatigue, loss of confidence and self-esteem, feelings of guilt, inability to make decisions, lack of initiative, loss of attention and concentration, sleep disturbances (insomnia or hypersomnia), appetite disturbances, weight gain, modification of psychomotor activity, and recurrent thoughts of death. The symptoms are not caused by a substance or another medical condition [3–5].

To determine the severity of depressive symptoms, a number of depression rating scales are available. Montgomery-Asberg Depression Rating Scale, Hamilton Depression Scale, and Young Mania Rating Scale are clinician-administered scales. In addition, self-administered scales can be useful (Patient Health Questionnaire, Beck Depression Inventory, Zung Self-Rating Depression Scale, and Mood Disorder Questionnaire) [6, 7].

The treatment of MDD is based on pharmacotherapy, which includes numerous drugs with various structures and mechanisms of action.

The aim of this chapter is to review the literature, highlight important aspects regarding the main incriminated theories of depression and the side effects of agents used to treat MDD, and especially point out the most relevant details of the latest antidepressant drugs.

This chapter synthetizes the classic and modern features concerning the MDD pathophysiology and treatment, as well as the information about the newest antidepressants introduced in the therapy (desvenlafaxine, levomilnacipran, vilazodone, and vortioxetine), detailing the mechanism of action, pharmacokinetic aspects, their side effects, and benefits. The first two substances have similar mechanisms of action to existing medications, and the other two compounds are multimodal antidepressants, which combine SSRI activity with additional receptor activity.

2. Pathophysiology of depression

Literature data highlighted that the pathophysiological mechanisms involved in the manifestation of affective disorders are mediated by numerous neurotransmitters, such as norepinephrine, serotonin, dopamine, acetylcholine, gamma-aminobutyric acid, and glutamate. In order to explain the phenomena that occur in the depression, several theories have been issued depending on the neuro-mediators involved in the pathogenic links, responsible for the development of the behavioral disturbances [8].

Monoaminergic theory of depression postulates that depressive manifestations are caused by the lack of one or more of the three essential neuro-mediators (serotonin, dopamine, norepinephrine) from the central nervous system synapses. These areas are situated especially in the cortex of the frontal lobe (dorsolateral, prefrontal, and orbitofrontal), the self-processing headquarters. In these areas, regional atrophy and atrophic alterations were observed, following the stress associated with the hypothalamic-pituitary-adrenal axis [8, 9].

Different types of deficits modulate the characters of depression:

- Serotonin deficiency causes in particular: sadness and thoughts with mainly negative content [8].
- Noradrenaline deficiency is associated with the diminution of voluntary and involuntary motor behaviors: the patient speaks slowly, in a monotone voice with low intensity, as if his energy is exhausted at each joint; the mimic and the gestures diminish; the posture begins to sketch the defense; the limbs are brought down (the generalized flexion tendency or even the genital posture appears); the patient's mobility decreases; in the beginning, the gestures of social and family significance are not performed; and the patient lacks personal hygiene behavior [10, 11].
- Dopamine deficiency is manifested by anhedonia; the patient can no longer enjoy any of the things that previously used to cause pleasure. From the outset, it should be noted that the therapeutic response appears differently for the three components. Often, the first neuro-mediator involved in the response is norepinephrine. Serotonin responds a little bit later. The patient regains his motor skills, before the ideation has normalized. This situation, in which the patient has the power to practice negative thoughts, appears in the early weeks of antidepressant therapy onset and is responsible for the suicidal accidents that may occur [9]. In conclusion, people with inhibited depression should be closely monitored during the first 3 weeks after the therapy is established.

A therapeutic response consists of 50% alleviation of the symptoms following administration of the antidepressant medication. A small percentage of people may develop resistance to antidepressants (through lack of synthesis or transport or excess metabolism of one or more monoamines). These patients are recommended to either potentiation of the treatment or electroconvulsive therapy, as a solution for achieving remission of the depression.

In these conditions, the therapeutic targets of currently used antidepressant drugs are aimed at augmenting the monoaminergic deficiency at the synaptic level.

This response can be achieved by:

- The action on the receptor level
- The receptor stimulation through neuro-mediator release
- Inhibition of the reuptake pump or inhibition of the metabolism enzyme

There is also evidence for the involvement of other (secondary) systems in the pathogenesis of depression, with the participation of acetylcholine, somatostatin, leptin, substance P, thyrotropin-releasing hormone (TRH), **brain-derived neurotrophic factor** (BRNF), gamma-aminobutyric acid (GABA), and glutamate [12].

It should be underlined that the reduction of any monoaminergic neuro-mediator is accompanied by upregulation events that increase the reactivity to small amounts of monoamine: this could be the mechanism responsible for hyper-serotoninergic reactions (serotoninergic pseudo-syndrome) manifested at the beginning of the treatment, with monoaminergic augmentation in persons with serotonin deficiency.

3. Treatment of depression

This affective disorder, which has a very long evolution, is generally underdiagnosed and insufficiently treated, statistical data showing that currently only half of the persons affected by depression have undergone pharmacological or non-pharmacological treatment. Despite the fact that 80–90% of cases of depression can be successfully treated, this disease considerably affects the quality of life of both patient and his family.

It is particularly important to early diagnose depression and rapidly establish the appropriate therapy to reduce the consequences of this pathological condition on the general (physical and mental) status of the patient.

Management of depression is complex, including therapeutic lines with targeted action on associated organic pathology, psychotherapy with the final goal of rebalancing the patient [13]. The treatment of affective disorders is of long duration and individualized, involving an adequate cooperation between doctor, patient, and his family for the choice of the appropriate antidepressant drug from a pharmacological and economical point of view.

Modern treatment of depression combines pharmacotherapy with alternative methods (represented by psychotherapy, hypnosis, cognitive behavioral treatment, interpersonal therapies). Short-term psychotherapeutic approaches, especially cognitive behavioral methods and interpersonal therapies, have been shown to be highly effective in relieving symptoms and diminishing the number of depressive episodes [14, 15]. More obvious results are obtained by combining psychotherapy with pharmacotherapy, which consists of the administration of antidepressants, their efficiency being demonstrated in 80% of depression cases. The pharmacodynamic effects of antidepressants occur after a period of time ranging from 2 to 4 weeks, during which psychotherapy has beneficial effects [16, 17].

It is known that in many cases the patients are rapidly discontinuing medication, conditions in which psychotherapy exhibits beneficial effects by increasing the patient's compliance/adherence, resulting in diminution or even elimination of the sense of isolation, as well as the powerless and hopeless feelings. These results improve communication with the patient, who becomes more conscious that stopping the administration of recommended drugs can lead to a recurrence of the disease. There are a lot of tools like questionnaires or patient-reported outcomes (PROs) that identify some different patterns of behavior of patients with depression with the aim of improving patients' adherence [18].

Depending on the clinical manifestations experienced by the patient (anxiety, insomnia, psychotic symptoms), antidepressant medication may be combined for limited periods of time with anxiolytic, sedative, or antipsychotic drugs. If affective disorders heavily respond to classical antidepressants, mood-stabilizing agents, electroconvulsive therapy, or bright light therapy may be associated.

3.1. Pharmacotherapy

A wide range of antidepressants are available nowadays, belonging to various therapeutic classes, with various mechanisms of action, effective in some affective disorders, but also a host of adverse effects as well as the possibility of interacting with other prescribed medications. In selecting the antidepressant, it is necessary to balance, on the one hand, its effectiveness in the affective disorder, and on the other hand, the adverse effects may occur (mild, moderate, severe, temporary, or lasting).

Table 1 summarizes the adult doses and some side effects of selected antidepressants (seizures and conduction abnormalities are dose-dependent side effects) [19].

Some of the antidepressant medication side effects may be unpleasant, others are dangerous to the patient, and they should be reported to the physician, who will decide to replace the drug or to adjust the dose. It is necessary to mention that, apart from specific adverse reactions, all antidepressants present a risk of suicide, especially at the beginning of treatment; therefore, the patient should be supervised and supported by family and entourage.

3.1.1. Classical antidepressants (first generation)

- Monoamine oxidase (MAO) inhibitors (MAOIs)

These agents inhibit the metabolism of monoamines (but not their synthesis) and release norepinephrine from postganglionic deposits (mebanazine, tranylcypromine, phenelzine) [20].

They have low selectivity, inhibiting other enzymes including dopamine-B-oxidase, diamine oxidase, amino acid decarboxylase, and choline dehydrogenase, which are responsible for some of the side effects of the group. Some of them act selectively for only one of the two MAO forms, the MAO-A: moclobemide, miaprine, pirlindole, and toloxatone [21]. The MAO-B inhibitors, such as selegiline and rasagiline, are reserved for Parkinson's disease therapy [22]:

- Irreversible, long-acting, noncompetitive inhibitors (phenelzine, tranylcypromine), of both MAO-A and MOA-B subtypes
- Reversible, short-acting, MAO-A selective inhibitors (moclobemide, brofaromine) that are experienced in Canada

MAOIs were among the first antidepressant drugs to be clinically introduced, which are used nowadays much less than other antidepressants because of their toxicity and serious drug and food interactions [23, 24].

For most of MAOIs, the enzyme blocking takes 2–6 weeks (new enzyme synthesis occurring only after 2 weeks) [25]. During this time, the administration of drugs that augment the monoamines' level (such as tricyclic antidepressants, fluoxetine, naphazoline, xylometazoline,

Drug	Initial dose (mg/day)	Usual dosage range (mg/day)	Side effects				
			Anticholinergic effects	Sedation	Orthostatic hypotension	Seizures	Conduction abnormalities
Amitriptyline	25	100–300	4+	4+	3+	3+	3+
Bupropion	150	150–300	+	0	0	4+	+
Citalopram	20	20–40	0	+	0	2+	2+
Desipramine	25	100–300	2+	2+	2+	2+	2+
Desvenlafaxine	50	50	+	+	0	2+	+
Doxepin	25	100–300	3+	4+	2+	3+	2+
Duloxetine	30	30-90	+	0	+	0	0
Escitalopram	10	10–20	0	0	0	0	0
Fluoxetine	20	20–60	0	0	0	2+	0
Fluvoxamine	50	50–300	0	+	0	2+	0
Imipramine	25	100–300	3+	3+	4+	3+	3+
Mirtazapine	15	15–45	+	2+	2+	0	+
Nefazodone	100	300–600	0	3+	3+	2+	+
Nortriptyline	25	50–150	2+	2+	+	2+	2+
Paroxetine	20	20–60	+	+	0	2+	0
Sertraline	50	50–200	0	0	0	2+	0
Trazodone	50	150–300	0	4+	3+	2+	+
Venlafaxine	37.5–75	75–225	+	+	0	2+	+

0, absent; +, very low; 2+, low; 3+, moderate; 4+, severe.

Table 1. Antidepressant drugs: adult doses and selected side effects [19].

or other drugs) or ingestion of food containing tyramine, the catecholamine precursor, can generate severe increase in blood pressure and death. In this situation, the intestinal fermented tyramine can be transported in blood and replaces norepinephrine in the vesicles, resulting in amplification the effects of the normal norepinephrine stimulation [26].

The main side effects of nonselective MAOIs are "cheese reaction" (severe hypertensive response to tyramine-containing foods, such as cheese, beer, wine, liver, sardines, well-hung meat, yeast, or soybean derivatives), anticholinergic side effects (dry mouth, blurred vision, urinary retention, etc.), postural hypotension, insomnia, weight gain, sexual side effects, convulsions (in overdose), and hepatotoxicity (rare). Nausea, insomnia, and agitation, but no "cheese reactions," were reported for moclobemide [19, 23].

- Tricyclic antidepressants are divided into subgroups with similar general structures:
  - Imipramine, desipramine, clomipramine, trimipramine, amitriptyline
  - Nortriptyline, butriptyline, doxepin, protriptyline [16]

- Tricyclic antidepressants have the following mechanisms of action:
  - Inhibition of serotonin transporter
  - Inhibition of norepinephrine transporter
  - Slight inhibition of dopamine reuptake
  - Stimulation 5-HT1A receptors
  - Inhibition of 5-HT2A receptors (but also affinity for 5-HT6 and 5-HT7 receptors)
  - Inhibition of alpha-1 receptors [27]

3.1.2. Heterocyclic antidepressants (second or third generation)

- With nonselective action on the amine neurotransmitters
- With anticholinergic effects (maprotilin, nomifensine, amoxapine)
- Without anticholinergic effects (venlafaxine, bupropion)
  - Heterocyclic antidepressants have the following mechanisms of action:
- Inhibition of alpha-2 receptors
- D2 receptor stimulation
- Inhibition of H1 receptors (for some compounds even H2 receptors)
- Inhibition of muscarine receptors
- Blockade of sodium and calcium channels (being responsible for cardiotoxicity) [16]

Various mechanisms of actions are responsible for the pharmacodynamic effects as well as for a lot of adverse effects, thus limiting their indications.

Adverse reactions are particularly due to the muscarine receptor blockade and consist of mucosal dryness, blurred vision, diminution of digestive tract motility, constipation, urinary retention, cognitive impairment and memory disturbances, increased body temperature, akathisia (psychological restlessness without physical agitation), tachycardia, hypotension, arrhythmias, and, in case of overdose, cardiotoxicity. Other side effects of tricyclic antidepressants include excessive sweating, paradoxical emotional changes (anxiety or the lack of emotional reactivity), modification in appetite and body weight, sexual dysfunction, muscle contraction, nausea and vomiting, and rarely rhabdomyolysis [16]:

- 5-HT2A/5-HT2C receptor antagonists (trazodone, nefazodone, mirtazapine)
- Selective serotonin reuptake inhibitors (SSRIs) (fluoxetine, sertraline, paroxetine, fluvoxamine, citalopram, escitalopram)

The onset of the therapeutic effect varies from a few hours to 2–3 days after SSRI administration. The peak blood concentration is reached in 10–21 days. Some of SSRIs persist for a long time in the body, for example, fluoxetine, which is completely eliminated only after 5 weeks [17, 28, 29].

During the treatment, the upregulation of the synapses can initially trigger a pseudo-serotoninergic syndrome, with psychomotor agitation, akathisia, insomnia, tremor, muscle fasciculation, fever, and vomiting. This syndrome is sensitive to benzodiazepine therapy, and usually the spontaneous resolution appears within a few days [16, 23].

Pure serotonin syndrome is particularly common for tricyclic antidepressants, more rarely for SSRIs, and most commonly occurs in drug combinations with metabolic inhibitors or with agents that may increase the serotonin level. Serotonin syndrome is manifested by agitation, confusion, excessive sweating, mydriasis, muscle spasms or muscle incoordination, fever, seizures, and coma.

The therapy with SSRIs is long-lasting, with the shortest treatment indicated being 3–6 months. As expected, a degree of dependence occurs; therefore, avoiding sudden discontinuation of treatment with SSRIs is essential. Otherwise insomnia, agitation, confusion, trembling, anxiety, and even hallucinatory phenomena may occur during treatment [30]:

- Mixed serotonin and norepinephrine reuptake inhibitors (SNRIs) (venlafaxine, desvenlafaxine, duloxetine, milnacipran, levomilnacipran)
- Dopamine and norepinephrine reuptake inhibitors (bupropion—reserved especially for asthenic and dopamine deficiency cases)
- Norepinephrine reuptake inhibitor (reboxetine)
- Serotonin disinhibitor and alpha-2 antagonists (mirtazapine)
- Serotonin antagonist and reuptake inhibitors (nefazodone, trazodone) [16, 23]

Among the antidepressant groups, SSRIs and SNRIs are preferred because not only of their therapeutic efficacy but also of the relatively small number and decreased severity of adverse effects [28, 30, 31].

4. Desvenlafaxine

The *O*-desmethylvenlafaxine or desvenlafaxine, a RS-4-[2-dimethylamino-1-(1-hydroxycyclohexyl)ethyl]phenol derivative, is the synthetic agent of the main active metabolite of venlafaxine. First of all, it was obtained as desvenlafaxine succinate (Pristiq®) and marketed by the company Wyeth Pharmaceuticals, which was subsequently acquired from the American corporation Pfizer [32]. This principal metabolite is 70% produced following the biodegradation of venlafaxine, the two drugs having similar demonstrated pharmacodynamic effects [33].

The development of desvenlafaxine was performed in hoping to improve the pharmacokinetic and clinical profile of the parent substance. It was approved as antidepressant drug by the FDA in February 2008, being available for medical use, in the treatment of MDD in adult patients, in May 2008 [34].

This agent was also experienced for the nonhormonal therapy of menopausal disorders associated by mild-to-serious vasomotor symptoms and in some types of anxiety [35, 36]. At the beginning of 2008, a product containing desvenlafaxine (Ellefore) was withdrawn from the market in the European Union, due to its insufficient documentation and clinical experience; but later in 2012, Pfizer corporation obtained the authorization for the use of Pristiq® in Spain. It also received the market authorization in Canada for the pharmacotherapy of depression in February 2009. A few years later, FDA approved the use of both brand and generic products containing desvenlafaxine fumarate (Desvenlafaxine fumarate, 2013) [37].

4.1. Pharmacological properties

In vitro studies revealed that desvenlafaxine determines the inhibition of serotonin and norepinephrine reuptake (10 times more potent for serotonin than for norepinephrine), thus blocking the removal of the main mediators (serotonin, norepinephrine) that affect mood, increasing their concentration at the synaptic level [32, 38]. No notable influence on muscarine, histamine, or alpha-1 adrenergic receptors and on the activity of monoamino oxidase was proven. Moreover, the lack of the influence on the functionality on sodium, potassium, chloride, or calcium ion channels was also evidenced [34, 39].

Dosage forms		50 mg, light-pink square pyramid extended-release tablet (containing 76 mg of desvenlafaxine succinate) 100 mg, reddish-orange square pyramid extended-release tablet (containing 152 mg of desvenlafaxine succinate)
Administration		Orally, once daily, with or without food
Dosage		Initial dosage of 50 mg, approximately at the same moment of time, each day, maintenance dose of 50 mg; the maximum accepted daily dose is 400 mg
Absorption		Not influenced by food intake
Time to maximum concentration		7.5 hours
Bioavailability		80% (being not influenced by the meals)
Protein-binding percentage		30%
T1/T2		Approximately 11 hours
Steady-state plasma concentrations		Achieved within 4–5 days after oral administration of a unique dose
Volume of distribution		3.4 L
Metabolism	Is mainly conjugated (via uridine 5′-diphospho-glucuronosyltransferase participation) and secondarily is metabolized by oxidation (through N-demethylation)	CYP3A4 CYP2D6 is not involved
Elimination		45% is eliminated and unchanged in urine, 72 hours after oral administration

Table 2. Pharmacological aspects of desvenlafaxine [32, 34, 38–41].

The drug is available as extended-release tablets for oral administration, which contain desvenlafaxine succinate (**Table 2**).

4.2. Side effects of desvenlafaxine

Current safety and efficacy information for the treatment of MDD highlights that most patients have well responded and tolerated and did not experience severe side effects to desvenlafaxine [42].

The most often described side effects of desvenlafaxine were nausea, vomiting, dry mouth, constipation, fatigue, headache, dizziness, insomnia, decreased appetite, hyperhidrosis, erectile dysfunction, and delayed ejaculation in men (**Table 3**) [34, 42].

Of these, the frequent adverse reactions, such as nausea, vomiting, dizziness, and headache, observed in short-term trials of up to 8 weeks in patients treated with desvenlafaxine (Pristiq®, Wyeth), usually lead to discontinuation of the treatment. The other side effects of the desvenlafaxine were related to the drug-drug interactions or to the presence of liver or kidney dysfunctions [38, 43].

4.3. Differences between desvenlafaxine and venlafaxine

Literature data highlighted some pharmacological differences between these two antidepressant drugs, but the therapeutic experience did not reveal substantial advantages of desvenlafaxine over venlafaxine use in the treatment of MDD.

System and organ	Manifestations
Cardiovascular	Palpitations, hypertension, tachycardia, hot flushes, orthostatic hypotension, peripheral coldness
Hematologic	Abnormal bleeding
Gastrointestinal	Nausea, vomiting, dry mouth, constipation, diarrhea, increase in transaminase levels
Nervous system	Dizziness, headache, insomnia, somnolence, tremor, paresthesia, dysgeusia, disturbance in attention, tinnitus, vertigo, depersonalization, hypomania, syncope, withdrawal syndrome, anxiety, abnormal dreams, nervousness, seizures, convulsions, extrapyramidal symptoms, serotonin syndrome
Genitourinary	Urinary hesitation, proteinuria, decreased libido, anorgasmia, anorgasmia, abnormal orgasm, erectile dysfunction, delayed ejaculation, ejaculation disorders in men, ejaculation failure
Respiratory	Yawning, epistaxis, interstitial lung disease, eosinophilic pneumonia
Skin	Hyperhidrosis, rash
Musculoskeletal	Musculoskeletal stiffness
Metabolic and endocrine	Decreased weight, increased blood cholesterol, decreased appetite, increased blood triglycerides, increased blood prolactin, hyponatremia
Others	Hypersensitivity reactions, fatigue, feeling jittery, blurred visions, mydriasis

Table 3. The most frequent adverse effects of desvenlafaxine [34, 38, 42, 44–46].

Preclinical and clinical investigations argue that venlafaxine and desvenlafaxine are basically equivalent, from the pharmacological point of view, even if there were observed dissimilarities, regarding especially the pharmacokinetic profile, dose regimen, and the drug interactions.

The most important differences between venlafaxine and desvenlafaxine are the following:

- Both antidepressant drugs present the similar mechanism of action, consisting of inhibition of serotonin and norepinephrine reuptake, but the desvenlafaxine's binding affinity at norepinephrine reuptake pumps is higher than venlafaxine's; yet this effect did not prove a therapeutic relevance [47].
- The clinical trials communicated similar tolerability and comparable incidence of adverse effects in patients treated for depression [48, 49]. Different clinical trials, performed during 8 weeks, revealed the superior efficacy of 100 and 400 mg, but not of 200 mg of desvenlafaxine (Pristiq®, Wyeth), on the improvement of depression symptomatology, clinically evidenced and assessed using Hamilton Depression Scale, and also the effectiveness of 400 mg on the remission rates, compared to placebo [36, 45, 50–52].
- The parent substance, venlafaxine, undergoes primarily biodegradation by the CYP 2D6-mediated oxidative reactions, to be converted into O-desmethylvenlafaxine, while desvenlafaxine is mainly inactivated by glucuronidation and secondarily metabolized by oxidation (through N-demethylation) to N,O-didesmethylvenlafaxine, its biodegradation being not influenced by the enzymatic system of cytochromes P450 (CYP 2D6) [40, 41]. Taking into account these issues, it was suggested that desvenlafaxine may be an advantageous option in patients with genetic polymorphisms of CYP2D6 (such as poor metabolizers) [34].
- As a result of the fact that desvenlafaxine has no markedly effect on CYP2D6, at therapeutic doses, it has lower risk of drug interactions, compared to venlafaxine, being preferred to prevent possible drug-drug interactions with CYP2D6 substrates (e.g., SSRIs, tricyclic antidepressants, several beta-blockers, quinidine, opioids). However, there are inconsistent evidences that desvenlafaxine would be more effective, better tolerated, or safer than venlafaxine in clinical use [40, 41, 44, 50].
- On the other hand, the treatment with desvenlafaxine may have a benefit, in terms of simpler dosage regimen compared with venlafaxine (small initial dose and lower minimum therapeutic dose), with more anticipated drug levels [45]. The FDA recommendations mention the indication of using the same 50 mg starting, and maintenance doses, for the treatment with desvenlafaxine, while the administration of extended-release form of venlafaxine needs titration from the starting dose of 37.5 mg per day to the maintenance dose of 150–225 mg per day [51]. The practical aspect is related to the fact that desvenlafaxine dosage choosing is based on the experience gained from several 8-week acute-phase clinical studies, but the real therapeutic response is not generally obtained in this short interval of time [34].

5. Levomilnacipran

Levomilnacipran, a (1S,2R)-2-(aminomethyl)-N,N-diethyl-1-phenylcyclopropane-1-carboxamide derivative, is the levo-enantiomer (1S, 2R-milnacipran) of racemate milnacipran, approved in 2009 for the treatment of fibromyalgia [53, 54]. It was discovered by Pierre Fabre Laboratories, France, and coproduced by Forest Laboratories, Inc. (Fetzima™), being approved by the FDA to be used for the treatment of MDD in adult patients in the United States and Japan in July 2013 and in Canada in May 2015 [55, 56]. It is not available on the market in the European Union and Australia.

The researches performed in laboratory animals showed that levomilnacipran is the pharmacologically more active enantiomer of the racemic mixture milnacipran, having 50, respectively, and 13 times more intense inhibitory activity on the norepinephrine and serotonin reuptake pumps, a higher peak blood concentration and a prolonged elimination half-life compared with the other enantiomer 1S,2R-milnacipran (coded F2696) [56–59].

Currently, it is under clinical research as a therapy of anxiety, bipolar disorders, post-traumatic stress diseases, vasomotor symptoms associated with menopause, peripheral neuropathy (especially associated with diabetes mellitus), and chronic musculoskeletal pain. Levomilnacipran has also been investigated for the treatment of fibromyalgia and phantom limb syndrome but was not approved to be used for these purposes [56].

5.1. Pharmacological properties

In vitro studies revealed that levomilnacipran determines the strong and selective inhibition of serotonin and norepinephrine reuptake transporters (two times more potent and selective for norepinephrine than for serotonin), with a consequent increasing of these mediator concentration in the central nervous system [60]. It proved to have a more balanced reuptake of both serotonin and norepinephrine compared to other known SNRIs [56, 61]. Due to this difference in the selectivity action on these neurotransmitters, it was postulated that levomilnacipran may be beneficial in MDD related to the norepinephrine deficiency, with the demonstrated improvement of core symptoms and, consequently, the patient social and occupational activities [62–64]. It may also be useful in refractory depression or in the cases susceptible to potential increase of weight gain during chronic therapy with other antidepressant drugs [61].

Levomilnacipran provides a "two and a half" action, the inhibition of the norepinephrine transporter facilitating the action of dopamine, as long as this mediator diffuses through the synapses, without requiring the presence of a transporter. No important activity on dopamine, serotonin (5-HT1–5-HT7), muscarine, histamine, and alpha- or beta-adrenergic and opioid receptors and no inhibitory effects on the monoamino oxidase were evidenced. The lack of affinity on the sodium, potassium, chloride, or calcium ion channels was also observed [56].

Recent researches highlighted the inhibitory action of levomilnacipran on the beta-site amyloid precursor protein cleaving enzyme-1, known to be responsible for the formation of β-amyloid plaque, thus arguing its possible use in the treatment of Alzheimer's disease [64].

The drug is available as extended-release capsules for oral administration, which contain levomilnacipran hydrochloride (**Table 4**).

5.2. Side effects of levomilnacipran

Short-term safety clinical trials revealed that most patients with MDD have well responded and tolerated and did not experience important side effects to levomilnacipran [62, 65]. The most common side effects of levomilnacipran were nausea, vomiting, hyperhidrosis, heart rate increase, tachycardia, palpitations, urinary hesitation, erectile dysfunction, and ejaculate disorders in men (**Table 5**) [56].

Long-term clinical studies documented that levomilnacipran manifested acceptable tolerability compared to placebo. Severe adverse reactions, such as nausea, vomiting, headache, tachycardia, hypertension, extrasystoles, and convulsion, observed in long-term trials of 48 weeks in patients treated with levomilnacipran, generally lead to discontinuation of the treatment. The other side effects of the levomilnacipran were related to the drug-drug interactions (inhibitors of CYP3A4 such as clarithromycin, ketoconazole, or itraconazole will increase its blood level) or to a concomitant hepatic, renal, and cardiac pathology. On the contrary, the association of levomilnacipran with the inducers of CYP3A4, such as rifampicin or carbamazepine, may determine a diminution of its plasma concentration [66, 67].

Dosage forms	20 mg, extended-release capsule with yellow cap and white body 40 mg, extended-release yellow-opaque capsule 80 mg extended-release capsule with pink cap and white body 120 mg, pink-opaque extended-release capsule
Administration	Orally, once daily, with or without food
Dosage	Initial dosage of 20 mg in a unique daily administration for 2 days, then increasing the dose to 40 mg per day; the maximum accepted daily dose is 120 mg
Absorption	Not influenced by food intake
Time to maximum concentration	6–8 hours
Bioavailability	92%
Protein-binding percentage	22%
T1/T2	Approximately 12 hours
Mean apparent total clearance	21–29 L/hour
Volume of distribution	387–473 L
Metabolism	Hepatic (primarily by CYP3A4); is converted primarily to two inactive metabolites: desethyl levomilnacipran and p-hydroxy-levomilnacipran with a minor involvement of CYP2C8, CYP2C19, CYP2D6, and CYP2J2
Elimination	58% of uncharged drug is excreted in the urine

Table 4. Pharmacological aspects of levomilnacipran [55, 56].

System and organ	Manifestations
Cardiovascular	Palpitations, tachycardia, hypertension, hot flushes, orthostatic hypotension, angina pectoris, supraventricular/ventricular extrasystoles
Hematologic	Abnormal bleeding
Gastrointestinal	Nausea, vomiting, constipation, sweeting, elevations in serum aminotransferase levels
Nervous system	Dizziness, headache, sleep troubles, excessive happiness or irritability, reckless behavior, nervousness, anxiety, difficulty concentrating, memory changes, confusion, weakness tremor, paresthesia disturbance in attention, drowsiness, dizziness, suicidal ideation, withdrawal syndrome, hallucinations, serotonin syndrome, seizures, convulsions, extrapyramidal symptoms, encephalopathy
Genitourinary	Urinary hesitation, decreased libido, erectile dysfunction, ejaculation disorders in men, ejaculation failure, delayed ejaculation, testicular pain
Respiratory	Upper respiratory tract infection
Skin	Hyperhidrosis, rash
Musculoskeletal	Musculoskeletal stiffness
Metabolic and endocrine	Decreased appetite, hyponatremia
Others	Hypersensitivity reactions, fatigue, blurred visions, visual disturbances, mydriasis, eye pain, swelling or redness in or around the eye

Table 5. The most frequent adverse effects of levomilnacipran [68–71].

Various preclinical researches showed the most intense antidepressant effect of levomilnacipran without substantially influencing the animal spontaneous locomotor activity, compared to other antidepressant drugs (venlafaxine, duloxetine) in different experimental animal models of depression, anxiety, and stress (such as forced swim test, tail suspension test, shock-induced ultrasonic vocalization) [70].

Short-term clinical trials highlighted the superior efficacy of levomilnacipran on depressive and disability symptoms (especially motivation and energy), and functional improvement of the patient status, compared to placebo, was quantified using the Montgomery-Asberg Depression Rating Scale, respectively, and the Sheehan Disability Scale. Significant superiority to placebo was also demonstrated by improvement of the patient's social activity, work, and family life [71–74]. On the other hand, there were insufficient and irrelevant data, regarding the efficacy for the relapse prevention in the long-term use of levomilnacipran [75].

5.3. Differences between levomilnacipran and milnacipran

Literature data indicated some pharmacological differences between these two antidepressant drugs, but the performed clinical studies did not prove considerable advantages of levomilnacipran over milnacipran use in the treatment of MDD.

There are few clinically relevant differences between levomilnacipran and milnacipran consisting of the simplicity of dose regimen, a more selective pharmacodynamic activity, an improved pharmacokinetic profile (with less complex correlation between blood concentration and the pharmacodynamic effect), and a reduced potential for drug interactions [76, 77].

The most important levomilnacipran's advantage is its once-daily administration of a sustained-release capsule compared with the twice-daily administration tablets of milnacipran, thus improving the patient's compliance especially to chronic therapy.

6. Vilazodone

Vilazodone, 2-benzofurancarboxamide, 5-[4-[4-(5-cyano-1*H*-indol-3-yl)butyl]-1-piperazinyl]-, hydrochloride (1:1) [78], is a new multimodal antidepressant drug indicated in the United States for the treatment of MDD in adult patients [79]. Its discovery program began in the mid-1990s, and FDA approved it in January 2011. It also received market authorization in Mexico and Canada for MDD pharmacotherapy. Moreover, it was found that vilazodone improves psychic and somatic symptoms in generalized anxiety disorder [80–82].

6.1. Pharmacological properties

Vilazodone is an indolalkylamine with a dual mechanism of action which consists of 5-HT1A receptor partial agonist and SSRI activity. It does not bind to the norepinephrine or dopamine reuptake sites with the same high affinity [81, 83].

The most prevalent out of the 14 different structurally distinct types of 5-HT receptors in the brain is 5-HT1A, which is localized especially in the raphe nuclei (presynaptic), the hippocampus, the frontal cortex, the dorsal horn of the spinal cord, the lateral septum, and the amygdala (postsynaptic). Presynaptic 5-HT1A receptors exhibit a key role in the pathophysiology and treatment of depression and anxiety disorders. According to Sahli et al., vilazodone is 60 times more selective for the 5-HT1A receptor than buspirone (the only 5-HT1A receptor partial agonist approved as an antidepressant) and has a SSRI activity 30 times more potent than fluoxetine (the first SSRI approved by FDA for MDD therapy) [83].

The drug is available as tablets for oral administration which contain vilazodone hydrochloride (**Table 6**).

6.2. Benefits versus adverse effects

Due to its unique mechanism of action, vilazodone has the potential benefits of faster onset of action, greater efficacy, and lower adverse event risks compared with currently used antidepressants, especially lower sexual side effects [84, 85]. Preclinical studies and clinical trials showed that vilazodone exhibits a diminished incidence of sexual adverse effects and minimal weight gain, similar for vilazodone and placebo, important aspects given that patients find sexual dysfunction, weight gain, and drowsiness to be the most frequently unpleasant adverse effects induced by antidepressants [86].

Sexual dysfunction was reported in 40–70% of SSRI-treated patients [87], and SSRIs therapy can determine sexual dysfunction in all three phases of the human sexual response cycle

Dosage forms		10 mg pink, film-coated, oval tablet 20 mg orange, film-coated, oval tablet 40 mg blue, film-coated, oval tablet
Administration		Orally, once daily, with food
Dosage		Initial dosage of 10 mg for 7 days, augment to 20 mg, the dose may be raised up to 40 mg after at least 7 days between dosage increases
Absorption Tmax		4–5 hours
Peak plasma concentration		156 ng/ml
Half-life		Approximately 25 hours
Absolute bioavailability		72% (with food)
Percentage of protein binding		96–99%
Metabolism	CYP pathways	CYP3A4 (primarily), CYP2C19, CYP2D6
	Non-CYP pathways	Carboxylesterase
Elimination		Unchanged drug (1% in the urine and 2% in the feces)
Common adverse reactions (>5%)		Diarrhea, nausea, vomiting, and insomnia
Drug interactions	CYP3A4 inhibitors	Vilazodone dose should be ≤ 20 mg once daily
	CYP3A4 inducers	Augment vilazodone dosage by twofold, over 1 to 2 weeks (up to 80 mg once daily) when coadministered with strong CYP3A4 inducers for more than 14 days

Table 6. Pharmacological aspects of vilazodone [19, 78, 83].

(desire, arousal, and orgasm). SSRI-induced sexual side effects cannot only reduce patients' quality of life but also cause treatment noncompliance and discontinuation, therefore augmenting the risk of MDD relapse and recurrence [88].

The effects of vilazodone (20 or 40 mg/day) on sexual functioning were also evaluated in healthy, sexually active adults assessed using the Changes in Sexual Functioning Questionnaire (CSFQ—a self-report questionnaire with 14 items used in antidepressant trials); vilazodone proved no significant effect on sexual functioning in healthy adults [87].

In a rat sexual behavior model, acute, sub-chronic, and chronic vilazodone treatment did not cause sexual dysfunction; moreover, 1 week vilazodone administration normalized sexual function in animals which registered paroxetine-induced sexual dysfunction [88].

Another benefit of this drug is related to its effect on anxiety disorder, and studies are being conducted to assess its efficacy in generalized anxiety disorder, post-traumatic stress syndrome, and social anxiety illness [80]. As Khan et al. reported, 8-week vilazodone therapy has led to improvements in four psychic anxiety items (anxious mood, depressed mood, tension, intellectual) and five somatic anxiety items (somatic muscular, somatic sensory, respiratory, cardiovascular, and autonomic symptoms) [82].

System and organ	Manifestations
Gastrointestinal	Nausea, vomiting, diarrhea, dry mouth
Nervous system	Dizziness, headache, insomnia
Cardiovascular	Chest pain, hypertension, tachycardia, palpitations, orthostatic hypotension
Others	Fatigue

Table 7. The most frequent adverse effects of vilazodone [81, 89].

Thus, vilazodone could be beneficial for some subgroups of patients, like ones with depression and comorbid anxiety, and patients with sexual side effects on SSRIs or other antidepressant drugs [85].

The results of the research published so far have shown that vilazodone has a relatively high level of safety and tolerability in adults. The most frequent adverse effects, which were related to the sleep quality and gastrointestinal tract, were transient in nature and mild to moderate in severity (**Table 7**) [80, 81, 85].

The adverse events occurred within the first few weeks of the therapy and led to few premature discontinuations [84, 89]. Further studies are needed not only to evaluate the efficacy and tolerability profile of vilazodone in the elderly and in adolescents with MDD but also to estimate its long-term safety. Due to the lack of information in human trials, it may be administered in pregnant women and lactation only if the benefits outweigh the potential risks [83–85].

Yet some results require further research on larger groups of subjects, with different characteristics, and for longer periods of time. Yan Li et al. developed a preclinical study and registered that vilazodone diminished depression-like behavior without altering visuospatial memory after 1 month of therapy. But after 3 months of treatment, vilazodone did not alter depression-like behavior or cognition. The drug was administered in therapeutic doses in healthy middle-aged female mice, which were assessed in the forced swim test (for depression-like behavior), in novel object recognition test (for recognition memory), or in novel object placement test (for visuospatial memory). The findings support the age difference in drug response for some antidepressant drugs [90].

7. Vortioxetine

Vortioxetine, 1-[2-(2,4-dimethyl-phenylsulfanyl)-phenyl]-piperazine, hydrobromide [91], is another new multimodal antidepressant drug that has been approved for MDD therapy in adult patients, in September 2013 in the United States, in December 2013 in European Union, and later in Canada, South Africa, Australia, Mexico, and South Korea [80].

Besides its antidepressant properties proven in several short-and long-term studies [93], vortioxetine demonstrated pro-cognitive effects in preclinical studies, affecting learning and memory processes (enhancing hippocampal synaptic plasticity and augmenting the output of pyramidal cells) [80, 94]. Positive results on cognitive function (memory and executive functioning) were also highlighted in clinical trials [92].

7.1. Pharmacological properties

Vortioxetine is a 5-HT3, 5-HT7, and 5-HT1D receptor antagonist, a 5-HT1B receptor partial agonist, a 5-HT1A receptor agonist, and an inhibitor of the serotonin transporter. It enhances 5-HT (more than a SSRI), NE, DA, acetylcholine, and HA levels in rat brain regions associated with MDD (like the PFC and the ventral hippocampus). Furthermore, it increases glutamatergic neurotransmission, probably through inhibiting GABA interneurons [80, 92, 94].

Its discovery program origins in the hypothesis were derived from researches of combined serotonin transporter inhibition and 5-HT1A receptor modulation; subsequently, the profile was modified toward a combination of serotonin transporter inhibition, 5-HT1A receptor agonistic activity, and 5-HT3 receptor antagonism [95].

The drug is available as immediate-release tablets for oral administration which contain the beta-polymorph of vortioxetine hydrobromide (**Table 8**).

Dosage forms		5 mg pink, almond-shaped biconvex film-coated tablet 10 mg yellow, almond-shaped biconvex film-coated tablet 15 mg orange, almond-shaped biconvex film-coated tablet 20 mg red, almond-shaped biconvex film-coated tablet
Administration		Orally, once daily, without regard to meals
Dosage		Initial dosage is 10 mg, augment to 20 mg/day, as tolerated consider 5 mg/day for patients who do not tolerate higher doses 5–10 mg/day therapy can be discontinued abruptly
Absorption Tmax		7–11 hours
Volume of distribution		Approximately 2600 L
Half-life		Approximately 66 hours
Absolute bioavailability		75% (unaffected by food)
Percentage of protein binding		98%
Metabolism	CYP pathways	CYP2D6 (primarily), CYP3A4/CYP3A5, CYP2C9, CYP2C19, CYP2C8, CYP2A6, CYP2B6
Elimination		59% in the urine and 26% in the feces, as metabolites
Common adverse reactions (>5%)		Nausea, constipation, and vomiting
Drug interactions	CYP2D6 inhibitors	Diminish vortioxetine dose by half when a strong CYP2D6 inhibitor is associated
	CYP inducers	Augment vortioxetine dose when a strong CYP inducer is coadministered for more than 14 days (up to no more than three times the original dose)

Table 8. Pharmacological aspects of vortioxetine [91, 96, 97].

7.2. Benefits versus adverse effects

Sanchez et al. reviewed preclinical studies and clinical trials and concluded that vortioxetine is different from SSRI and SNRI antidepressants on the strength of its multimodal mechanism of action, both inhibition of the potent serotonin transporter and direct modulation of 5-HT receptors [95].

Studies evaluating the drug have shown the following benefits:

- There are no necessary dose adjustments in patients with mild to moderate renal or hepatic impairment or on the basis of patient age, sex, and race. Yet its efficacy and safety have not been sufficiently studied in children or adolescents, and it is not approved for pediatric patients; nevertheless, some recent results in acute therapy are promising [91, 96–98].
- Cognitive dysfunction is often present in MDD, and a pro-cognitive effect of an antidepressant is an important issue. Rosenblat et al. reported in a systematic review and meta-analysis that of the antidepressants evaluated (vortioxetine, duloxetine, paroxetine, citalopram, phenelzine, nortriptyline, and sertraline), vortioxetine appeared to have the largest effect size on psychomotor speed, executive control, and cognitive control [99]. Pehrson et al. reviewed the preclinical data for vortioxetine's effects, at clinically relevant doses, on cognitive function in mechanistic assays and in animal models of depression. The results suggest its neurogenesis and plasticity-promoting effects and that it may have advantages over other antidepressant drugs (regarding its effects on cognitive function) [100].
- Vortioxetine exhibited improvement in overall functioning for patients with MDD and high anxiety symptoms, which often co-occurs; frequently, these patients are difficult to treat, with a higher risk of side effects and suicidal ideation, and register a slower response [93, 97, 101].
- Due to its relatively long half-life, vortioxetine presents a low risk of discontinuation symptoms after rapid cessation of the administration [95, 97].
- Vortioxetine therapy had a low incidence of worrisome changes in vital signs, electrocardiogram parameters, and advantages when talking about treating symptoms of MDD in the elderly [95, 97].
- Unlike most currently antidepressants, drug-associated weight gain and sexual side effects (decreased/loss of libido, delayed ejaculation, erectile dysfunction, anorgasmia, ejaculation disorder, disturbance in sexual arousal, orgasmic sensation decreased/anorgasmia, abnormal orgasm, sexual dysfunction, and ejaculation failure) were not significantly different from placebo [95, 97].

Vortioxetine was well tolerated both in short-term and in long-term studies. Mild to moderate nausea was the most commonly registered side effect, and its frequency was dose related [95, 102]. Due to the lack of well-controlled studies, its administration in pregnancy and lactation is not recommended (**Table 9**) [91].

With more than 50 antidepressant drugs available worldwide (most of them approved for more than 10 years), vortioxetine is the newest agent and needs to determine its place in MDD therapy [97].

System and organ	Manifestations
Gastrointestinal	Nausea, diarrhea, dry mouth, constipation, vomiting, flatulence
Nervous system	Dizziness, abnormal dreams
Skin	Pruritus

Table 9. The most frequent adverse effects of vortioxetine [91, 96, 97, 103].

8. Conclusion

A wide range of antidepressant drugs are available on the market, the most frequent used being the SSRIs, but they do not represent the ideal medication to treat MDD, especially due to the various side effects, that considerably influence the patient's daily life and activity.

Recently introduced in therapy, the four new antidepressants have demonstrated a number of benefits compared to classical medication, represented by faster onset of pharmacodynamic effects, simpler dosage regimen, without necessity of dose adjustment, slight superior efficacy, and less importantly short-term side effects.

Although they have proven efficacy in treating MDD and are being investigated for other possible indications, the risk that these drugs may cause adverse effects following prolonged administration is not fully elucidated. And since most patients undertake antidepressant therapy for several months or years and may suffer from various comorbidities, future detailed clinical trials are needed to establish the pharmaco-toxicological profile of these new antidepressants.

Author details

Maria Bogdan[1*†], Eliza Gofita[1], Daniela Cornelia Calina[1], Adina Turcu-Stiolica[1], Anca Oana Docea[1], Tudor Adrian Balseanu[2], Adrian Camen[3], Gratiela Eliza Popa[4], Gabriela Rusu[5], Ina Cristofor[5], Liliana Pavel[6] and Liliana Mititelu-Tartau[5†]

*Address all correspondence to: bogdanfmaria81@yahoo.com

1 Faculty of Pharmacy, University of Medicine and Pharmacy of Craiova, Romania

2 Faculty of Medicine, University of Medicine and Pharmacy of Craiova, Romania

3 Faculty of Dental Medicine, University of Medicine and Pharmacy of Craiova, Romania

4 Faculty of Pharmacy, "Gr. T. Popa" University of Medicine and Pharmacy Iasi, Romania

5 Faculty of Medicine, "Gr. T. Popa" University of Medicine and Pharmacy Iasi, Romania

6 Faculty of Medicine, "Dunarea de Jos" University of Medicine and Pharmacy Galati, Romania

† These authors contributed equally.

References

[1] Gotlib I, Hammen C. Handbook of Depression. New York: Guilford Press; 2002

[2] Murray ED, Buttner N, Price BH. Depression and psychosis in neurological practice. In: Bradley WG, Daroff RB, Fenichel GM, Jankovic J, editors. Neurology in Clinical Practice. 6th ed. Philadelphia, PA: Butterworth Heinemann; 2012

[3] American Psychiatric Association: Diagnostic and Statistical Manual of Mental Disorders, 5th ed. Arlington, VA: American Psychiatric Association; 2013. pp. 155-188

[4] Belmaker RH, Agam G. Major depressive disorder. New England Journal of Medicine. 2008;**358**(1):55-68

[5] Mondimore FM. Depression, The Mood Disease. Baltimore: The Johns Hopkins University Press; 2006

[6] Cvetkovich A. Depression: A Public Feeling. Durham, NC: Duke University Press Books; 2012

[7] Teter CJ, Kando JC, Wells BG. Major Depressive Disorder. In DiPiro JT, Talbert RL, Yee GC, Matzke GR, Wells BG, Posey LM, editors. Pharmacotherapy: A Pathophysiologic Approach. 8th ed. USA: McGraw Hill Medical; 2011. pp. 1173-1190

[8] Reis S, Grenyer BF. Pathways to analitic and introjective depression. Psychol Psychother. 2002;**75**:445-459

[9] Krishnan V, Nestler EJ. The molecular neurobiology of depression. Nature. 2008;**455**(7215):894-902

[10] Maletic V, Robinson M, Oakes T, Iyengar S, Ball SG, Russell J. Neurobiology of depression: An integrated view of key findings. International Journal of Clinical Practice. 2007;**61**(12):2030-2040

[11] Delgado PL, Moreno FA. Role of norepinephrine in depression. Journal of Clinical Psychiatry. 2000;**61**(Suppl. 1):5-12

[12] Calabrese F, Molteni R, Racagni G, Riva MA. Neuronal plasticity: A link between stress and mood disorders. Psychoneuroendocrinology. December 2009;**34**(Suppl. 1): S208-S216

[13] Arroll B, Elley CR, Fishman T, Goodyear-Smith FA, Kenealy T, Blashki G, Kerse N, Macgillivray S. Antidepressants versus placebo for depression in primary care. The Cochrane Database of Systematic Reviews. 2009;**3**:CD007954

[14] Gartlehner G, Hansen RA, Morgan LC, Thaler K, Lux L, Van Noord M, Mager U, Thieda P, Gaynes BN, Wilkins T, Strobelberger M, Lloyd S, Reichenpfader U, Lohr KN. Comparative benefits and harms of second-generation antidepressants for treating major depressive disorder: An updated meta-analysis. Annals of Internal Medicine. 2011;**155**(11): 772-785

[15] Fineberg NA, Brown A, Reghunandanan S, Pampaloni I. Evidence-based pharmacotherapy of obsessive-compulsive disorder. The International Journal of Neuropsychopharmacology. 2012;**15**(8):1173-1191

[16] Katsung BG, Trevor, A.J. Basic & Clinical Pharmacology. 13th ed. McGrow Hill Education, Lange; 2015. Section V, Chapter 30

[17] Fournier JC, DeRubeis RJ, Hollon SD, Dimidjian S, Amsterdam JD, Shelton RC, Fawcett J. Antidepressant drug effects and depression severity: A patient-level meta-analysis. Journal of the American Medical Association. 2010;**303**(1):47-53

[18] Turcu-Stiolica A, Taerel AE, Turcu-Stiolica R. Identifying and measuring compliance and adherence in antidepressing taking. Procedia Economics and Finance. 2014;**15**:836-839

[19] Teter CJ, Kando JC, Wells BG. Major Depressive Disorder. In DiPiro JT, Talbert RL, Yee GC, Matzke GR, Wells BG, Posey LM, editors. Pharmacotherapy: A Pathophysiologic Approach, 9th ed. USA: McGraw Hill Medical; 2014. pp. 1047-1066

[20] Fangmann P, Assion HJ, Juckel G, González CA, López-Muñoz F. Half a century of antidepressant drugs: On the clinical introduction of monoamine oxidase inhibitors, tricyclics, and tetracyclics. Part II: Tricyclics and tetracyclics. Journal of Clinical Psychopharmacology. February 2008;**28**(1):1-4

[21] Thase ME. MAOIs and depression treatment guidelines. Journal of Clinical Psychiatry. 2012;**73**(7):e24

[22] Grady MM, Stahl SM. Practical guide for prescribing MAOIs: Debunking myths and removing barriers. CNS Spectrums. 2012;**17**:17

[23] Rang HP, Ritter JM, Flower RJ, Henderson G. Antidepressant drugs. In Hyde M. (Ed): Rang and Dale's Pharmacology. 8th ed. UK: Elsevier; 2016. pp. 570-584

[24] O'Donnell JM, Shelton RC. Drug therapy of depression and anxiety disorders. In Brunton LL, Chabner BA, Knollmann BC, editors. Goodman & Gillman's The Pharmacological Basis of Therapeutics. 12thh ed. USA: McGraw Hill Medical; 2011. pp. 397-416

[25] Shulman KI, Herrmann N, Walker SE. Current place of monoamine oxidase inhibitors in the treatment of depression. CNS Drugs. 2013;**27**(10):789-797

[26] McCabe-Sellers BJ, Staggs CG, Bogle ML. Tyramine in foods and monoamine oxidase inhibitor drugs: A crossroad where medicine, nutrition, pharmacy, and food industry converge. Journal of Food Composition and Analysis. 2006;**19**:S58-S65

[27] Gillman PK. Tricyclic antidepressant pharmacology and therapeutic drug interactions updated. British Journal of Pharmacology. 2007;**151**(6):737-748

[28] Preskorn SH, Ross R, Stanga CY. Selective serotonin reuptake inhibitors. In: Preskorn SH, Feighner HP, Stanga CY, Ross R, editors. Antidepressants: Past, Present and Future. Berlin: Springer; 2004. pp. 241-262

[29] Gibbons RD, Hur K, Brown CH, Davis JM, Mann JJ. Benefits from antidepressants: Synthesis of 6-week patient-level outcomes from double-blind placebo-controlled randomized trials of fluoxetine and venlafaxine. Archives of General Psychiatry. 2011;**69**(6): 572-579

[30] Jakobsen JC, Katakam KK, Schou A, Hellmuth SG, Stallknecht SE, Leth-Møller K, Iversen M, Banke MB, Petersen IJ, Klingenberg SL, Krogh J, Ebert SE, Timm A, Lindschou J, Gluud C. Selective serotonin reuptake inhibitors versus placebo in patients with major depressive disorder. A systematic review with meta-analysis and trial sequential analysis. BMC Psychiatry. 2017;**17**(1):58

[31] Stahl SM, Grady MB. SNRIs: Their pharmacology, clinical efficacy, and tolerability in comparison with other classes of antidepressants. CNS Spectrums. 2005;**10**(9):732-747

[32] Pristiq (desvenlafaxine) leaflet available from the FDA website https://www.accessdata.fda.gov/drugsatfda_docs/label/2012/021992s030lbl.pdf

[33] Lemke TL, Williams DA, Roche VF, Zito SW. Foye's Principles of Medicinal Chemistry. 7th ed. Lippincott Williams and Wilkins. Philadelphia, PA: Wolters Kluwer; 2013. pp. 570-630

[34] Colvard MD. Key differences between Venlafaxine XR and Desvenlafaxine: An analysis of pharmacokinetic and clinical data. Mental Health Clinician. 2014;**4**(1):35-39

[35] Thase ME, Kornstein SG, Germain JM, Jiang Q, Guico-Pabia C, Ninan PT. An integrated analysis of the efficacy of desvenlafaxine compared with placebo in patients with major depressive disorder. CNS Spectrums. 2009;**14**(3):144-154

[36] Soares CN, Kornstein SG, Thase ME, Jiang Q, Guico-Pabia CJ. Assessing the efficacy of desvenlafaxine for improving functioning and well-being outcome measures in patients with major depressive disorder: A pooled analysis of 9 double-blind, placebo-controlled, 8-week clinical trials. Journal of Clinical Psychiatry. 2009;**70**(10):1365-1371

[37] VandenBerg AM. What's new? Isomers, metabolites and prodrugs, oh my! Mental Health Clinician. January 2014;**4**(1):1-1

[38] Pae CU. Desvenlafaxine in the treatment of major depressive disorder. Expert Opinion on Pharmacotherapy. 2011;**12**(18):2923-2928

[39] Nichols AI, Behrle JA, Parks V, Richards LS, McGrory SB, Joel Posener J, Patat A, Paul J. Pharmacokinetics, pharmacodynamics, and safety of desvenlafaxine, a serotonin-norepinephrine reuptake inhibitor. Journal of Bioequivalence & Bioavailability. 2013;**5**:022-030

[40] Nichols AI, Focht K, Jiang Q, Preskorn SH, Kane CP. Pharmacokinetics of venlafaxine extended release 75 mg and desvenlafaxine 50 mg in healthy CYP2D6 extensive and poor metabolizers: A randomized, open-label, two-period, parallel-group, crossover study. Clinical Drug Investigation. 2011;**31**(3):155-167

[41] Lobello KW, Preskorn SH, Guico-Pabia CJ, Jiang Q, Paul J, Nichols AI, et al. Cytochrome P450 2D6 phenotype predicts antidepressant efficacy of venlafaxine: A secondary

analysis of 4 studies in major depressive disorder. Journal of Clinical Psychiatry. 2010;**71**(11):1482-1487

[42] Clayton AH, Kornstein SG, Rosas G, Guico-Pabia C, Tourian KA. An integrated analysis of the safety and tolerability of desvenlafaxine compared with placebo in the treatment of major depressive disorder. CNS Spectrums. 2009;**14**(4):183-195

[43] Patroneva A, Connolly SM, Fatato P, Pedersen R, Jiang Q, Paul J, Guico-Pabia C, Isler JA, Burczynski ME, Nichols AI. An assessment of drug-drug interactions: The effect of desvenlafaxine and duloxetine on the pharmacokinetics of the CYP2D6 probe desipramine in healthy subjects. Drug Metabolism & Disposition. December 2008;**36**(12): 2484-2491

[44] Boyer P, Montgomery S, Lepola U, Germain JM, Brisard C, Ganguly R, et al. Efficacy, safety, and tolerability of fixed-dose desvenlafaxine 50 and 100 mg/day for major depressive disorder in a placebo-controlled trial. International Clinical Psychopharmacology. 2008;**23**(5):243-253

[45] Liebowitz MR, Manley AL, Padmanabhan SK, Ganguly R, Tummala R, Tourian KA. Efficacy, safety, and tolerability of desvenlafaxine 50 mg/day and 100 mg/day in outpatients with major depressive disorder. Current Medical Research and Opinion. 2008; **24**(7):1877-1890

[46] Baird-Bellaire S, Behrle JA, Parker VD, Patat A, Paul J, Nichols AI. An open-label, single-dose, parallel-group study of the effects of chronic hepatic impairment on the safety and pharmacokinetics of desvenlafaxine. Clinical Therapeutics. June 2013;**35**(6): 782-794

[47] Bymaster FP, Dreshfield-Ahmad LJ, Threlkeld PG, Shaw JL, Thompson L, Nelson DL, et al. Comparative affinity of duloxetine and venlafaxine for serotonin and norepinephrine transporters in vitro and in vivo, human serotonin receptor subtypes, and other neuronal receptors. Neuropsychopharmacology. 2001;**25**(6):871-880

[48] Deecher DC, Beyer CE, Johnston G, Bray J, Shah S, Abou-Gharbia M, et al. Desvenlafaxine succinate: A new serotonin and norepinephrine reuptake inhibitor. Journal of Pharmacology and Experimental Therapeutics. 2006;**318**(2):657-665

[49] Alipour A. STEPS for cost-effective prescribing of serotonin-norepinephrine reuptake inhibitors (SNRIs) in major depressive disorder: Focus on venlafaxine (Effexor®) versus duloxetine (Cymbalta®). Mental Health Clinic. 2013;**3**(4):100

[50] DeMartinis NA, Yeung PP, Entsuah R, Manley AL. A double-blind, placebo-controlled study of the efficacy and safety of desvenlafaxine succinate in the treatment of major depressive disorder. Journal of Clinical Psychiatry. 2007;**68**(5):677-688

[51] Septien-Velez L, Pitrosky B, Padmanabhan SK, Germain J-M, Tourian KA. A randomized, double-blind, placebo-controlled trial of desvenlafaxine succinate in the treatment of major depressive disorder. International Clinical Psychopharmacology. 2007; **22**(6):338-347

[52] Rosenthal JZ, Boyer P, Vialet C, Hwang E, Tourian KA. Efficacy and safety of desvenlafaxine 50 mg/d for prevention of relapse in major depressive disorder: A randomized controlled trial. Journal of Clinical Psychiatry. 2013;**74**(2):158-166

[53] Mease PJ, Clauw DJ, Gendreau RM, Rao SG, Kranzler J, Chen W, Palmer RH. The efficacy and safety of milnacipran for treatment of fibromyalgia: A randomized, double-blind, placebo-controlled trial. Journal of Rheumatology. 2009;**36**:398-409

[54] Clauw DJ, Mease P, Palmer RH, Gendreau RM, Wang Y. Milnacipran for the treatment of fibromyalgia in adults: A 15-week, multicenter, randomized, double-blind, placebo-controlled, multiple-dose clinical trial. Clinical Therapeutics. 2008;**30**:1988-2004

[55] Fetzima (levomilnacipran) leaflet available from the FDA website https://www.accessdata.fda.gov/drugsatfda_docs/label/2017/204168s004lbl.pdf

[56] Asnis GM, Henderson MA. Levomilnacipran for the treatment of major depressive disorder: A review. Neuropsychiatric Disease and Treatment. 2015;**11**:125-135

[57] Zadka Ł, Dziwota E, Olajossy M. Levomilnacipran – A successor of milnacipran with a higher noradrenergic selectivity. Acta Poloniae Pharmaceutica. 2016;**73**:285-289

[58] Bakish D, Bose A, Gommoll C, Chen C, Nunez R, Greenberg WM, Liebowitz M, Khan A. Levomilnacipran ER 40 mg and 80 mg in patients with major depressive disorder: A phase III, randomized, double-blind, fixed-dose, placebo-controlled study. Journal of Psychiatry & Neuroscience. January 2014;**39**(1):40-49

[59] Citrome L. Levomilnacipran for major depressive disorder: A systematic review of the efficacy and safety profile for this newly approved antidepressant – What is the number needed to treat, number needed to harm and likelihood to be helped or harmed? International Journal of Clinical Practice. November 2013;**67**(11):1089-1104

[60] Bradley AJ, Lenox-Smith AJ. Does adding noradrenaline reuptake inhibition to selective serotonin reuptake inhibition improve efficacy in patients with depression? A systematic review of meta-analyses and large randomised pragmatic trials. Journal of Psychopharmacology (Oxford). 2013;**27**(8):740-758

[61] Sansone RA, Sansone LA. Serotonin norepinephrine reuptake inhibitors: A pharmacological comparison. Innovations in Clinical Neuroscience. 2014;**11**(3-4):37-42

[62] MacAluso M, Kazanchi H, Malhotra V. Levomilnacipran for the treatment of major depressive disorder. Current Psychiatry. December 2013;**12**(12):50-52 54-55

[63] Mago R, Mahajan R, Thase ME. Levomilnacipran: A newly approved drug for treatment of major depressive disorder. Expert Review of Clinical Pharmacology. March 2014; **7**(2):137-145

[64] Rizvi SM, Shaikh S, Khan M, Biswas D, Hameed N, Shakil S. Fetzima (levomilnacipran), a drug for major depressive disorder as a dual inhibitor for human serotonin transporters and beta-site amyloid precursor protein cleaving enzyme-1. CNS & Neurological Disorders – Drug Targets. 2014;**13**(8):1427-1431

[65] Gommoll CP, Greenberg WM, Chen C. A randomized, double-blind, placebo-controlled study of flexible doses of levomilnacipran ER (40-120 mg/day) in patients with major depressive disorder. Journal of Drug Assessment. 2014;**3**:10-19

[66] O'Donnell JM, Shelton RC. Pharmacotherapy of depression and anxiety disorders. In: Brunton LL, Chabner BA, Knollman BC, editors. Goodman & Gilman. The Pharmacological Basis of Therapeutics. 12th ed. New York: McGraw-Hill; 2011. pp. 397-416

[67] Sambunaris A, Bose A, Gommoll CP, Chen C, Greenberg WM, Sheehan DV. A phase III, double-blind, placebo-controlled, flexible-dose study of levomilnacipran extended-release in patients with major depressive disorder. Journal of Clinical Psychopharmacology. 2014;**34**:47-56

[68] Reuben A, Koch DG, Lee WM, Acute Liver Failure Study Group. Drug-induced acute liver failure: Results of a U.S. multicenter, prospective study. Hepatology. 2010;**52**:2065-2076

[69] Saraceni MM, Venci JV, Gandhi MA. Levomilnacipran (Fetzima): A new serotonin-norepinephrine reuptake inhibitor for the treatment of major depressive disorder. Journal of Pharmacy Practice. 2013;**27**:389-395

[70] Auclair AL, Martel JC, Assié MB, Bardin L, Heusler P, Cussac D, Marien M, Newman-Tancredi A, O'Connor JA, Depoortère R. Levomilnacipran (F2695), a norepinephrine-preferring SNRI: Profile in vitro and in models of depression and anxiety. Neuropharmacology. July 2013;**70**:338-347

[71] Scott LJ. Levomilnacipran extended-release: A review of its use in adult patients with major depressive disorder. CNS Drugs. November 2014;**28**(11):1071-1082

[72] Montgomery SA, Mansuy L, Ruth AC, Li D, Gommoll C. The efficacy of extended-release levomilnacipran in moderate to severe major depressive disorder: Secondary and post-hoc analyses from a randomized, double-blind, placebo-controlled study. International Clinical Psychopharmacology. 2014;**29**:26-35

[73] Blum SI, Tourkodimitris S, Ruth A. Evaluation of functional health and well-being in patients receiving levomilnacipran ER for the treatment of major depressive disorder. Journal of Affective Disorders. 2015;**170**:230-236

[74] Bruno A, Morabito P, Spina E, Muscatello MR. The role of levomilnacipran in the management of major depressive disorder: A comprehensive review. Current Neuropharmacology. 2016;**14**(2):191-199

[75] Shiovitz T, Greenberg WM, Chen C, Forero G, Gommoll CPA. randomized, double-blind, placebo-controlled trial of the efficacy and safety of levomilnacipran ER 40-120mg/day for prevention of relapse in patients with major depressive disorder. Innovations in Clinical Neuroscience. 2014;**11**:10-22

[76] Chen L, Greenberg WM, Gommoll C, O'Connor J, Zukin SR, Periclou A, Ghahramani P. Levomilnacipran pharmacokinetics in healthy volunteers versus patients with major depressive disorder and implications for norepinephrine and serotonin reuptake inhibition. Clinical Therapeutics. September 2015;**37**(9):2059-2070

[77] Puozzo C, Panconi E, Deprez D. Pharmacology and pharmacokinetics of milnacipran. International Clinical Psychopharmacology. 2002;**17**(Suppl. 1):S25-S35

[78] Viibryd (vilazodone) leaflet available from the FDA website https://www.accessdata.fda.gov/drugsatfda_docs/label/2015/022567s012lbl.pdf

[79] Papadakis MA, McPhee SJ. Current Medical Diagnosis & Treatment 2015. 54th ed. USA: McGraw Hill Education; 2015

[80] Dale E, Bang-Andersen B, Sanchez C. Emerging mechanisms and treatments for depression beyond SSRIs and SNRIs. Biochemical Pharmacology. 2015;**95**:81-97

[81] Shi L, Wang J, Xu S, Lu Y. Efficacy and tolerability of vilazodone for major depressive disorder: Evidence from phase III/IV randomized controlled trials. Drug Design, Development and Therapy. 2016;**10**:3899-3907

[82] Khan A, Durgam S, Tang X, Ruth A, Mathews M, Gommoll CP. Post hoc analyses of anxiety measures in adult patients with generalized anxiety disorder treated with vilazodone. Primary Care Companion for CNS Disorders. 2016;**18**(2):1-8

[83] Sahli Z, Banerjee P, Tarazi F. The preclinical and clinical effects of vilazodone for the treatment of major depressive disorder. Expert Opinion on Drug Discovery. 2016;**11**(5): 515-523

[84] Zhang XF, Wu L, Wan DJ, Liu RZ, Dong Z, Chen M, Yu SY. Evaluation of the efficacy and safety of vilazodone for treating major depressive disorder. Neuropsychiatric Disease and Treatment. 2015;**11**:1957-1965

[85] Hellerstein DJ, Flaxer J. Vilazodone for the treatment of major depressive disorder: An evidence-based review of its place in therapy. Core Evid. 2015;**10**:49-62

[86] Croft HA, Pomara N, Gommoll C, Chen D, Nunez R, Mathews M. Efficacy and safety of vilazodone in major depressive disorder: A randomized, double-blind, placebo-controlled trial. Journal of Clinical Psychiatry. 2014;**75**(11):e1291-e1298

[87] Clayton A, Durgam S, Li D, Chen C, Chen L, Mathews M, Gommoll C, Szegedi A. Effects of vilazodone on sexual functioning in healthy adults: Results from a randomized, double-blind, placebo-controlled and active-controlled study. International Clinical Psychopharmacology. January 2017;**32**(1):27-35

[88] Oosting R, Chan J, Olivier B, Banerjee P. Vilazodone does not inhibit sexual behavior in male rats in contrast to paroxetine: A role for 5-HT1A receptors? Neuropharmacology. 2016;**107**:271-277

[89] Croft HA, Pomara N, Gommoll C, Chen D, Nunez R, Mathews M. Efficacy and safety of vilazodone in major depressive disorder: A randomized, double-blind, placebo-controlled trial. Journal of Clinical Psychiatry. November 2014;**75**(11):e1291-e1298

[90] Li Y, Sanchez C, Gulinello M. Distinct antidepressant-like and cognitive effects of antidepressants with different mechanisms of action in middle-aged female mice. International Journal of Neuropsychopharmacology. 2017;**20**(6):510-555

[91] Brintellix (vortioxetine) leaflet available from the FDA website https://www.accessdata.fda.gov/drugsatfda_docs/label/2013/204447s000lbl. pdf

[92] Caraci F, Leggio GM, Salomone S, Drago F. New drugs in psychiatry: Focus on new pharmacological targets. F1000Research. 2017;**30**(6):397

[93] Florea I, Loft H, Danchenko N, Rive B, Brignone M, Merikle E, Jacobsen PL, Sheehan DV. The effect of vortioxetine on overall patient functioning in patients with major depressive disorder. Brain and Behavior. February 2, 2017;**7**(3):e00622

[94] Bortolato B, Miskowiak KW, Köhler CA, Maes M, Fernandes BS, Berk M, Carvalho AF. Cognitive remission: A novel objective for the treatment of major depression? BMC Medicine. January 22, 2016;**14**:9

[95] Sanchez C, Asin KE, Artigas F. Vortioxetine, a novel antidepressant with multimodal activity: Review of preclinical and clinical data. Pharmacology & Therapeutics. January 2015;**145**:43-57

[96] Brintellix (vortioxetine) leaflet available from the EMA website http://www.ema.europa.eu/docs/en_GB/document_library/EPAR_-_Product_Information/human/002717/WC500159449.pdf

[97] Kelliny M, Croarkin PE, Moore KM, Bobo WV. Profile of vortioxetine in the treatment of major depressive disorder: An overview of the primary and secondary literature. Therapeutics and Clinical Risk Management. August 12, 2015;**11**:1193-1212

[98] Findling RL, Robb AS, DelBello M, Huss M, McNamara N, Sarkis E, Scheffer R, Poulsen LH, Chen G, Lemming OM, Areberg J, Auby P. Pharmacokinetics and safety of vortioxetine in pediatric patients. Journal of Child and Adolescent Psychopharmacology. August 2017;**27**(6):526-534

[99] Rosenblat JD, Kakar R, McIntyre RS. The cognitive effects of antidepressants in major depressive disorder: A systematic review and meta-analysis of randomized clinical trials. International Journal of Neuropsychopharmacology. July 25, 2015;**19**(2):1-13

[100] Pehrson AL, Leiser SC, Gulinello M, Dale E, Li Y, Waller JA, Sanchez C. Treatment of cognitive dysfunction in major depressive disorder–a review of the preclinical evidence for efficacy of selective serotonin reuptake inhibitors, serotonin-norepinephrine reuptake inhibitors and the multimodal-acting antidepressant vortioxetine. European Journal of Pharmacology. April 15, 2015;**753**:19-31

[101] Baldwin DS, Florea I, Jacobsen PL, Zhong W, Nomikos GG. A meta-analysis of the efficacy of vortioxetine in patients with major depressive disorder (MDD) and high levels of anxiety symptoms. Journal of Affective Disorders. December 2016;**206**:140-150

[102] Schatzberg AF, Blier P, Culpepper L, Jain R, Papakostas GI, Thase ME. An overview of vortioxetine. Journal of Clinical Psychiatry. December 2014;**75**(12):1411-1418

[103] Meeker AS, Herink MC, Haxby DG, Hartung DM. The safety and efficacy of vortioxetine for acute treatment of major depressive disorder: A systematic review and meta-analysis. Systematic Reviews. March 1, 2015;**4**:21